DAOIST REFLECTIONS
FROM SCHOLAR SAGE

DAOIST REFLECTIONS
FROM SCHOLAR SAGE

Damo Mitchell and his students

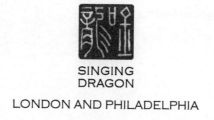

SINGING
DRAGON

LONDON AND PHILADELPHIA

First published in 2017
by Singing Dragon
an imprint of Jessica Kingsley Publishers
73 Collier Street
London N1 9BE, UK
and
400 Market Street, Suite 400
Philadelphia, PA 19106, USA

www.singingdragon.com

Library of Congress Cataloging in Publication Data
Names: Mitchell, Damo, author.
Title: Daoist reflections from scholar sage / Damo Mitchell and his students.
Description: Philadephia : Singing Dragon, 2016. | Includes bibliographical
 references and index.
Identifiers: LCCN 2016017574 | ISBN 9781848193215 (alk. paper)
Subjects: LCSH: Taoism.
Classification: LCC BL1920 .M58 2016 | DDC 181/.114--dc23 LC record
available at https://urldefense.proofpoint.com/v2/url?u=https-3A__lccn.loc.
gov_2016017574&d=BQIFAg&c=euGZstcaTDllvimEN8b7jXrwqOf-v5A_
CdpgnVfiiMM&r=VCKr2NBFNTs4O_kp07esGY2J-doQEb4zTq5sCaeXa-I&m=z8QI
IloOwbBlulh1MUhNetaYbucQ9kkYxzPUZn7WdQw&s=KdKE9W9N7SiOE3rElu4L
sR-AzUmeW8Ypj_Ugkz9QtE0&e=

British Library Cataloguing in Publication Data
A CIP catalogue record for this book is available from the British Library

ISBN 978 1 84819 321 5
eISBN 978 0 85701 274 6

Printed and bound in Great Britain

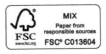

CONTENTS

PREFACE

An important aspect of any traditional study is exploration of the underlying theory. For many practitioners of Daoism this can seem like a strange statement; this is because it is generally seen as a purely 'doing' tradition. Whilst it is true that all aspects of the practice must be directly experienced, this should always be supported by the foundation of our cognitive understanding. In this way our intellectual mind and our body-consciousness can come together to lead us along the path of Daoism. This was the original reason why I began to write.

In the beginning I was simply writing for myself, a way of structuring my thoughts. As I wrote it helped me to crystallise my understanding of Daoism. This continued for some time until I naturally moved into writing more publicly. Initially this writing was in the form of several books, but alongside this the idea for the Scholar Sage online magazine was born. This was a platform for me to write about various aspects of Daoism; sometimes technical aspects and sometimes purely theoretical. As much as anything it was a way for me to continue writing without being caught up in lengthy explorations of a single topic as is generally the case when you are writing a book. With the Scholar Sage project I could jump about from subject to subject as well as 'fill in the blanks' with regards to small pieces of information that just had no obvious place within a larger text.

The website quickly proved popular and started to grow. On top of this it started to attract more writers from within the school and I was pleasantly surprised by two things: first, there were a number of people willing and able to write for the public and, second, they really knew their subject! I would like to be able to take credit for their knowledge due to me being their primary teacher, but actually I am pretty sure that they are so knowledgeable about the internal arts because they are highly motivated people who train diligently and then support this practice with theoretical study.

The site continues to grow and now includes a video section as well. It is exciting to see the positive feedback we get from readers who are happy to have a free source of information. Compared with many other Eastern traditions, Daoism is still relatively hard to find many writings on beyond almost incomprehensible translations of classics, which are only really for those deep in the more advanced aspects of the tradition.

The only real negative feedback we have received with regards to Scholar Sage is that many people do not like reading articles on the screen of their computer. Time and again people have asked us to produce a hard copy of the articles that they can hold in their hands, and so here it is: the Scholar Sage book!

What I have done is go through the site and select the most popular articles from the last couple of years and put them into this book. The majority of the articles are by me, but there are also articles written by other teachers in our school as well as senior students. It is always an amazing thing to sit and read articles by other teachers and students in the school. The level of effort and passion they have put into their practice shines out from their writings, as does the skill level they demonstrate in their chosen arts. I wish I could have selected more articles from the site as many of them were excellent, but if I did this the book would end up the size of a phone directory! Instead I selected some of my favourite articles as well as those I feel give a good spread of information on the topic of Daoism. Thank you so much to the other writers in the school who were happy to have their work contributed to this book.

Please note that the nature of the book means there is a variety of articles covering different subjects. I primarily tried to select articles on Nei Gong and alchemy, since this is what most people will have encountered in my previous writings, but there are also a couple of articles on martial arts and some relevant to Chinese medicine as well. In order to try and smooth out any continuity issues in the book I have gone back and re-edited the articles somewhat. This has been to minimise any repeated information in the book. As I edited the articles I also found that I felt the need to add sections to them, so you will also notice that several of the articles are longer and more in depth than the version you may have read online at the Scholar Sage website.

On top of this there are a few articles in here that never appeared on the site.

I hope that this book provides some new information for readers, as well as sometimes being thought provoking and, who knows, maybe even entertaining! The Scholar Sage website is stacked full of all sorts of esoteric guidance and I feel that this book is a reflection of the site. Consequently, there is a whole jumble of instructions and information to dive into. I hope you enjoy it.

Damo Mitchell, Vilamoura, Portugal

NOTES ON THE TEXT

Throughout this book we have used the Pinyin system of Romanisation for the majority of Chinese words. Please note that much of the theory in this book differs greatly from Western science. The classical Chinese approach to understanding the organs of the body, for example, is based around the function of their energetic system rather than their physical anatomy. To distinguish the two understandings from each other we have used capitalisation to indicate the Chinese understanding of the term. 'Heart' refers to the classical Chinese understanding of the organ, whilst 'heart' refers to the physical organ as understood within contemporary Western biological sciences.

As well as this we have had a lot of correspondence from native Chinese speakers who have been reading our books. This, combined with an increase in Chinese students, means that it is wise for us to put the Chinese characters next to each Pinyin term that we use within our writing. In order to not 'overcrowd' the text we have included the Chinese character the first time each Pinyin term is used. The only exception to this is if it seems relevant to include the Chinese character on another occasion such as when listing Pinyin terms. As well as this, there is a full glossary of Chinese terminology at the rear of this book.

Also note that this book has contributions from a number of different authors. Though all of these writers are members of the same school, it is inevitable that they will each have their own take on the subject material. This means that there may occasionally be contradictions between different writers as each has their own opinion. Rather than detracting from the book, we feel that it makes the book more interesting! Also we have tried to edit the writings a little to make sure that the same terminology is used throughout; that being said, there may be some slight differences in the way that the terminology is used from person to person.

ACKNOWLEDGEMENTS

First and foremost, thank you to all of the writers who have contributed their work to this book. Thanks to my father Paul Mitchell, my partner Roni Edlund, Tino Faithfull, Lauren Faithfull, Rob Aspell, Linda Hallett, Ellie Talbot, Seb Smith, Kulsoom Shah, Donna Pinker and Richard Agnew.

On top of this, many thanks to those writers who have contributed to the Scholar Sage online magazine as well as the many readers who have also contributed their suggestions for articles. Apologies that our writing speed is not up to completing all of the articles we are regularly asked to write!

A big thanks to those who helped with the editing of this book: Jason (Sam) Smith, Lauren Faithfull and Tino Faithfull.

Much gratitude to those who helped with some of the images: Joe Andrews, Spencer Hill, Roni Edlund and Jason Smith.

Finally, thanks very much to Jessica Kingsley and Singing Dragon for producing the seventh book directly related to the Lotus Nei Gong School of Daoist Arts!

1

THE DING AND THE LU
Damo Mitchell

The Ding (鼎) and the Lu (爐) are two important regions of the energy body utilised within Daoist alchemical meditation. The Ding is the 'cauldron', whilst the Lu is the 'furnace' or 'fire of cultivation'. When working with these aspects of our inner universe it is crucial that we develop an understanding of their location, their function and the process of awakening them. If we look at the various arts and practices that have come out of the Daoist tradition we can see that each has its own terminology and unique ways of working. Understanding the nature of the Ding and the Lu is important to alchemical meditation, whereas they are rarely discussed within less intricate practices such as Qi Gong (氣功).

The Ding is situated within the centre of the lower Dan Tien (丹田). Many think that the Ding is the lower Dan Tien itself but this is not the case. The lower Dan Tien is made up of numerous layers that can divide and rotate freely around each other like various layers on a gyroscope. This segmentation of the lower Dan Tien takes place as people move deeper into Nei Gong (內功) practice. It can be directly experienced as a series of individual rotations taking place within the lower abdomen. The size of the Dan Tien can also adjust according to the level of internal attainment of the practitioner. At highly developed stages it merges with the other energy centres of the body and the three separate Dan Tien are no more – only Dan Yuan (丹圓) exists, the microcosmic manifestation of Hundun (混沌), original chaos. Unlike the various outer layers of the lower Dan Tien, the Ding continues to exist until such a time that, according to classical teachings, the body is totally dissolved into light – a state known as the attainment of the 'diamond body' within ancient teachings. When a person has achieved the state of Dan Yuan it is said that their entire energetic and spiritual field rotates as one unified whole rather than in separate rotational pathways as is the case for the majority of living beings. Obviously such high states of accomplishment are rarely achieved in modern or indeed past times; on top of this there is the added limitation to many people's practice that their logical mind will not allow them to accept that such things are even possible.

The Ding is said to be roughly an inch in size for men, with a woman's Ding being slightly smaller (those Daoists are very exact people when they keep records). It is the key place within which Jing (精) is consolidated, Qi (氣) is converted and alchemically generated inner substances are immersed in order to 'rebirth' the spirit into its original state. This all takes place through controlled use of the breath and the Lu furnace. This process stimulates the Ding to generate an energetic catalyst for transformation.

Many of the esoteric teachings within Daoism are encoded within their architecture and artwork. Over the years as I have travelled to different temples and holy sites across Asia, I have taken the time to examine the artwork closely. Teachers can manifest in many different places, not just within people you meet. Ancient art and architecture is a gateway to the past if you know how to read it. Figure 1.1 is an example of the Ding and the Lu from Daoist Nei Dan (內丹) represented as a large metal cauldron. Anybody who has visited Chinese temples from the Daoist tradition is likely to have seen something very similar to this.

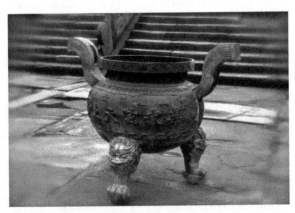

FIGURE 1.1: THE DING CAULDRON

The Ding is the body of the cauldron. These cauldrons are common in most Daoist temples and used to send offerings to the Heavens in the form of incense, magical offerings and even pretend money. They always stand upon three legs as shown. The number three represents the trinity of either: Jing, Qi and Shen (神); Body, Breath and Mind; or Heaven, Man and Earth. These are the three powers that must be brought together in order to complete the alchemical process within the Ding in order to generate alchemical change.

When Daoist monks or nuns burn their offerings of incense within the centre of the Ding it sends smoke up into the sky. This is the spirit of the offerings moving up towards the Heavenly immortal realm. Microcosmically this is manifested as the movement of the spiritual energies upwards into the 'Heaven' of the body, the pineal gland, and its energetic counterpart, the upper Dan Tien. This is the result of the correct and efficient usage of the Ding and the Lu.

Figure 1.2 shows the Ding on the right and the Lu on the left. The trigrams above the two symbols denote them as either extreme Yin (陰) or Yang (陽). The process of alchemical transformation relies on the two opposing powers of Yin and Yang being brought together to form an energetic union.

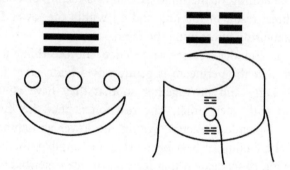

FIGURE 1.2: CLASSICAL DEPICTION OF DING AND LU

Within the body the Ding exists within the lower abdomen, as stated above, within the centre of the lower Dan Tien, whilst the Lu is the furnace that is essentially the energy around the region of the perineum. Figure 1.3 shows the physical location of the Ding and Lu within the body.

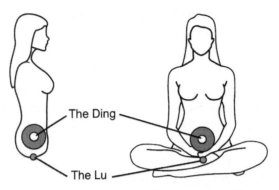

FIGURE 1.3: THE DING AND LU WITHIN THE BODY

Initially, when starting out within alchemical training, a practitioner will need to help the energy within the centre of the lower Dan Tien, the location of the Ding, to begin stirring. This is generally achieved through periods of silent sitting practice, with the awareness gently resting within this region of the body. It does not usually take very long for a practitioner to begin feeling the activity of the Jing and Qi within the region of the Ding. The resultant feeling is one of gentle heat within the lower abdominal region. This is generally accompanied by a gradual stilling of the mind as well as a feeling of contentment that is a direct result of the Jing and Qi within the lower Dan Tien having a stabilising effect upon the mind.

In the intermediate stages of practice, the breathing method is changed so that the perineum is gently raised upon inhalation. This brings the Ding and Lu together so that they have an energetic relationship with each other. The reaction is that the 'furnace' is lit and the alchemical reaction within the lower abdominal region increases. The feeling of heat becomes more tangible; there is also a clear sensation of movement that feels much like water bubbling, and thus the foundations for alchemical practice have been established.

Within the Daoist tradition, understanding the nature and location of the Ding and the Lu was key to initiating alchemical change as well as beginning the conversion of the three treasures of Jing, Qi and Shen.

If we compare various lines of teachings from within the Daoist tradition, we can see how different masters passed different methods on to their students. The variations in the methods being transmitted down through the generations within their school were largely due to the aims of their training. In contemporary Qi Gong schools, we can still see today two main models of understanding with regards to how the energetic system works. Each of these models provides a different conceptual outline of the Dan Tien locations. As a student in China I was initially confused by these differences of opinion, as I was training with teachers from both lines. Of course, each teacher claimed that they had the correct and true transmission whilst my other teachers were mistaken. It was only once I moved deep enough into the alchemical processes of Daoism that I began to develop an understanding of why these differences had manifested within each teacher's training. First, let us look at the two different models. Figure 1.4 shows the first and arguably most common model for the location of the three Dan Tien.

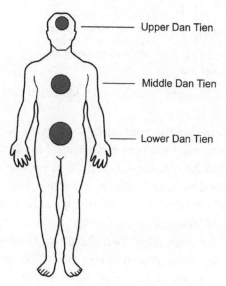

FIGURE 1.4: THE ENERGETIC MODEL

Here we have the lower Dan Tien situated, as stated above, within the lower abdomen. Its location will vary from person to person for various reasons. These can include such factors as individual body shape and size, age and even geographical location. This is because the human body is a direct microcosmic manifestation of our outer environment. With regards to the lower Dan Tien, this can be seen as being like the molten core of our planet whilst the equatorial line is manifested within our body as the Dai Mai (帶脈) or 'girdling meridian'. This meridian runs around our waist, as shown in Figure 1.5. It actually has several other minor branches, which are not depicted, but the main pathway of the meridian depicted is the line that has a direct relationship with both the equator and the lower Dan Tien.

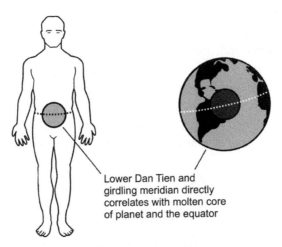

Lower Dan Tien and girdling meridian directly correlates with molten core of planet and the equator

FIGURE 1.5: THE EQUATOR, THE GIRDLING MERIDIAN AND THE DAN TIEN

People living closer to the equator or even on it will find that the lower Dan Tien actually sits further up within the body, whilst those living further from the equator will find the lower Dan Tien is situated lower down. This difference in distance is subtle, but as a person who travels extensively it is very clear to feel how the Dan Tien shifts if you are practising enough to be familiar with its general location. Directly below the lower Dan Tien should sit the perineum and an important meridian point known as Hui Yin (會陰). It is here that the alchemical Lu is situated. It is an important task for all practitioners of the internal arts to locate the lower Dan Tien early on in their practice, especially if the conceptual model shown in Figure 1.4 is the model used within your system.

The middle Dan Tien sits within the centre of the chest at the height of your heart. Microcosmically this energy centre corresponds to the energy of the sun in men and the moon in women. Nourishing this area of the energy body through directly bathing the chest in either sun or moonlight is a common spiritual practice of many traditions, including Daoism. This is the emotional centre as well as the place in which the mind and our Qi interact with one another.

The upper Dan Tien sits within the centre of the head, with the pineal gland being the physical anchor by which this energetic sphere attaches itself to the realm of manifestation.

I tend to refer to this common model of the three Dan Tien as the 'energetic model', as it tends to be used by Qi Gong and Nei Gong methods concerned with energetic movement, rotation and refinement. Commonly, practitioners are aiming to nourish the body with an increase of Qi from the environment, circulate it more effectively through the body and then finally refine it upwards so that it nourishes the consciousness. There may be a number of variations on this theme, but this tends to be the general theory behind those practices that utilise the 'energetic model'. It is common within medical Qi Gong as well as spiritual Qi Gong and many Nei Gong systems.

Figure 1.6 shows the second common model for understanding the location of the three Dan Tien.

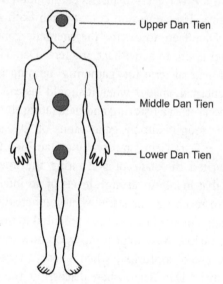

FIGURE 1.6: THE ALCHEMICAL MODEL

In this model, the lower Dan Tien is situated right on the perineum itself. It is much smaller than the lower Dan Tien is seen to be within the 'energetic model', and its location is non-variable from person to person. The middle Dan Tien is situated within the centre of the body. This is a region of the body commonly known as the 'yellow court' and it corresponds to a meridian point known as Zhong Wan (中脘).

If you wish to locate this area on yourself then measure four fingers' width from the upper border of your naval, as shown in Figure 1.7. This will get you roughly in the right region; now palpate around a little until you locate a slightly tender region of the body. In many people there is a slight depression to be found as well. The upper Dan Tien, like the previous model, is located within the centre of the head.

I refer to this as the 'alchemical model', as it is the view of the energy body commonly used by systems of practice greatly influenced by Daoist alchemy. Unlike pure Qi Gong methods, alchemy aims to work with far more subtle and refined aspects of the body's energetic substances. These 'substances' are drawn directly from the congenital region of our spiritual makeup. Practice at this level is complex and requires in-depth instruction to ensure that any success is achieved.

As I mentioned earlier, whichever model is being taught, it is common for the teacher to state that theirs is the correct model. The fact is that both are correct – it just depends upon what your aims are in the practice. The confusion comes when both models use the same term, the Dan Tien, to discuss the energetic conversion centres they are focusing upon. In actual fact, the term Dan Tien has become something of a general term for 'gathering, refining and circulating' regions of the energetic matrix when it should instead be referring to a specific function – that of storing and generating the 'Dan' (丹), the alchemical elixir sought out by generations of Daoist practitioners. If truth be told, a Dan Tien is not really a Dan Tien unless a person has actively reached the stage of generating the internal elixir, the alchemical pill that manifests at high levels of an internal alchemist's practice. Prior to reaching this stage what you actually have is just a Tien (田), an energetic field that has the potential to interact with Jing, Qi and Shen in various ways depending upon how you use them.

In order to avoid confusion, when I teach, I use the common names of the three Dan Tien when discussing the energy centres shown in the 'energetic model'. I then use the alternative, alchemical names for the centres shown within the 'alchemical model'. When put together what we have is the combined model shown in Figure 1.7. This is a model used within more esoteric systems of Daoist practices. These systems use a combination of Qi Gong, Nei Gong and Nei Dan in order to achieve their aims.

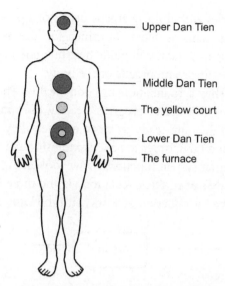

Upper Dan Tien

Middle Dan Tien

The yellow court

Lower Dan Tien

The furnace

FIGURE 1.7: THE COMBINED MODEL

In the combined model we can see that the lowest energetic centre is the Lu, the furnace. Above this is the lower Dan Tien, with the Ding, the cauldron, at its centre. Above the lower Dan Tien is the yellow court, and above this again is the middle Dan Tien. Situated within the centre of the head is the upper Dan Tien, the energetic centre agreed upon by almost all systems of practice.

With this model we can see how the Ding and the Lu interact with and function alongside the three Dan Tien.

The manner in which they work together will vary according to the stage a practitioner has reached. Within my personal teaching I generally take students through an early process using Qi Gong exercises, both moving and stationary. In this case the concerns are shifting energy through the body as well as purging the body of energetic toxins, a substance known as Xie Qi (邪氣) or 'sick energy/ information'. In order to do this, more energy is brought into the body via the lower Dan Tien and then circulated through various orbits known commonly as the 'microcosmic orbits' or the 'small water wheels'. The mind is calmed through deep rhythmic breathing and this helps to centre the middle Dan Tien. As the emotional centre starts to grow still, this changes the quality of the Qi being circulated.

It no longer carries with it the energetic debris of a person's emotional highs and lows. This is much healthier for the body, and with continued practice a person will guide healthier energetic information to the various channels and organs of the body.

This establishes a foundation in good health. This is important for a person if they wish to progress steadily onto more alchemical practices. When they are ready to move on then they begin to work with the Ding and Lu in order to generate transformation with regards to how the internal system functions. If we look at Figure 1.8 we can see how the body's energetic circulation via the three Dan Tien takes place prior to the introduction of work with the Ding and the Lu.

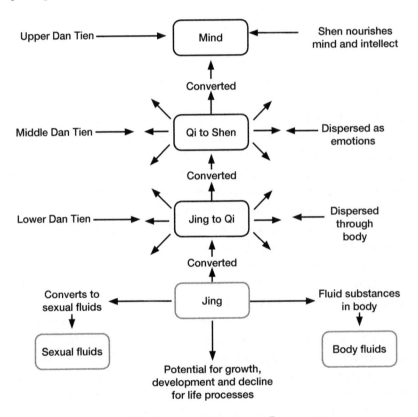

FIGURE 1.8: STANDARD ENERGETIC CIRCULATION

In this instance, the Jing, our essence, moves from the region of the Kidneys down towards the perineum where it starts to go through various natural processes. The first is the generation of body fluids, including the sexual fluids. The second is the continuation of our ageing process. The Jing carries within it a seed of information, a kind of inbuilt code if you like, that governs the speed and nature of how we age and eventually die. How fast we move through this process depends upon how efficiently we govern our inner processes and how well we look after our health. On top of this, of course, are natural strengths and weaknesses, which are an inherent part of all of us. The third function for Jing to carry out is conversion into Qi when it is combined with the air we breathe and the food we eat. Essentially, if we breathe effectively and eat healthy food then less Jing will be used in the creation of Qi but there will still always be a certain amount of our Jing being processed into Qi all of the time. This Qi moves upwards into the middle Dan Tien where it converts into Shen and nourishes our intellectual mind. It is for this reason that many Qi Gong practitioners find that their mind grows calmer and more capable with regards to problem solving and similar functions.

During this process we lose energy through dispersal and emotional movements. More than anything our emotional swings and extremes drain us of the Qi we are converting from Jing each second.

Through practices such as Qi Gong we help to make this process more efficient, and for many this can be life changing in itself. To be able to generate more energy within the body and feel more vitally charged and more centred in the mind is important on so many levels. Governing this process is the foundation of deeper work – alchemical work using the aspect of the energetic system shown within the 'alchemical model'. Once we introduce the Ding and the Lu we have the ability to convert the body's functioning to the process shown in Figure 1.9. This is the beginning of true alchemical change.

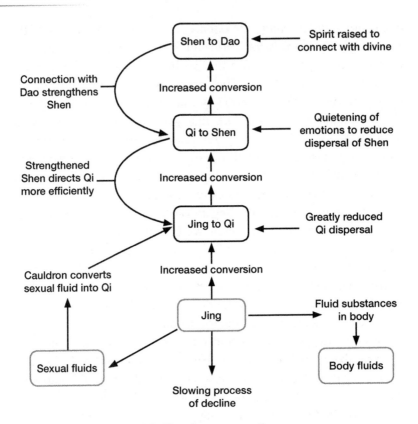

FIGURE 1.9: THE ALCHEMICAL CIRCULATION

Through a combination of guidance from a teacher and perseverance, a practitioner will be able to engage the process of the Ding and the Lu. As the Lu, the furnace, is 'lit', it starts to generate a change within the way that the Jing converts within the body. The interaction of the Lu with the Ding establishes the 'cauldron' of conversion within the centre of the lower Dan Tien, and in this way the energetic substances of the body begin to 'cook'. This changes the three processes of the Jing outlined above so that the following changes take place. First, the Jing still produces bodily fluids; this does not change. Second, the ageing process begins to slow down and in many cases even reverse; nothing too extreme (you won't become an infant again!), but it is common for thinning hair to become thicker and wrinkles on the face to fade away. It is within this process that the longevity of Daoist practitioners is to be found. It is true that even those who still live an average-length life tend to look a lot more youthful in their face than would be expected for their age. I will also let you in on a little secret here. Many people I met in China marvelled at the lack of grey hairs that their teachers had. Students would be amazed at 60–70-year-old teachers without even a single grey hair on their head. The truth is that a lack of grey hair is often seen as a hallmark of Qi Gong mastery, and consequently many Qi Gong masters in China dye their hair regularly so as to keep up the illusion! The third and most important change in the way that the Jing circulates is that more is converted upwards into Qi and this is added to by the essence contained within the sexual fluids. This essence is extracted by the actions of the Lu furnace and sent upwards to join the Jing being converted into Qi within the lower Dan Tien. The result of this is a far higher degree of vitality as well as a lessening of base sexual desires, which were previously generated by the spiritual actions of the sexual fluids. This is an important aspect of the training for many practitioners, as overcoming base desires is a serious hurdle to many internal processes.

The increased levels of Qi nourish the body to a far higher degree and this in turn generates a higher degree of Shen. Now instead of nourishing the intellectual mind, it invigorates a person's deeper underlying consciousness. This is vital for spiritual evolution, as a person's true nature can begin to grow whilst the acquired layers of the mind begin to become less dominant.

This process of transformation must take place for serious practitioners of the Daoist arts, as without this kind of work they will forever be stuck within the early, surface stages of their training. Of course, for many this is enough. For those who simply want a deeper level of relaxation and improved vitality, alchemical work is not required. But those who wish to understand the deeper layers of Daoist transformational practices must learn to govern and improve the efficiency of their internal processes. This largely requires understanding of the conceptual models of the Daoist energetic system as well as the use of the Ding and the Lu.

2

FIRE, WATER, DRAGON AND TIGER

Damo Mitchell

Within alchemical language the spiritual energies of the Heart and Kidneys are known respectively as the energies of Li (離) and Kan (坎). These are the two trigrams known as Fire and Water within the *Yi Jing* (*I Ching*) (易经). Li is formed from two solid lines with a broken Yin line within its centre; Kan is the opposite of Li and formed from two broken Yin lines surrounding a solid Yang line. These two symbols are shown in Figure 2.1. These are two of the key Gua (卦) or 'sacred symbols' from the *Yi Jing*.

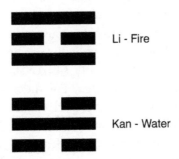

Li - Fire

Kan - Water

FIGURE 2.1: LI AND KAN – FIRE AND WATER

Within Qi Gong and Nei Gong practices, the merging of Fire and Water refers to bringing the Qi of the Heart and Kidneys into such a state whereby they can communicate with each other. Here there is an alchemical reaction between the two of them whereby the excitable function of the Heart's energy balances the more reserved energy of the Kidneys. This takes place on an energetic level and is accompanied by tangible sensations of Qi flow within the torso, which generate distinct reactions within the body.

The alchemical interaction of Fire and Water through Daoist meditative practices takes a slightly different form, as here we are discussing the mental/spiritual/psyche aspects of the Heart and Kidneys rather than their energy. In this case we are discussing the difference between the acquired mind and the congenital mind and the imbalances that have caused our consciousness to divide into two halves in the first place. Here the trigrams of Li and Kan can be discussed as follows.

Li has two Yang lines on the outside representing the virtuous nature of wisdom. Unfortunately, at the centre of these two lines sits a single broken Yin line representing the biases and acquired knowledge that is getting in the way of accessing or trusting our inherent wisdom.

Kan has two broken Yin lines representing mundane thoughts and trivial attachments. They are surrounding a single solid Yang line that represents the intuitive understanding of the nature of reality. We could access this intuitive knowledge (and indeed many people do on occasion) if only we could dig it out of the mundane thoughts that are burying it.

Philosophically, Fire is said to rise and Water to sink within the body. Since Fire sits above, at the level of the Heart, it is inevitable that it will blaze upwards, mostly fuelled by our emotional states, which cause it to move away from the Water energy, which it needs to mix with. Water sinks downwards, represented by the wastage of our essence that we do not adequately preserve throughout our lives. This causes it to move away from the Heart's energy, and in this way we divide these two forces even more. As they divide, they cause the ageing processes to hasten, and the formation of the acquired nature (sometimes called the ego) is sped up. Realisation is pulled even further away from us as our mundane thoughts and conditioned thinking overtakes us. The 'tool' of the mind has become the master of consciousness and thus elevation of spirit is denied to us. The separation of Fire and Water is shown in Figure 2.2.

In order to change this, through alchemy we must mix the energies of Fire and Water, which meet halfway at a location within the body known as the yellow court. If we are to get the two to meet with each other we must locate the Dragon and Tiger and get them to copulate. Alchemical language like this can be confusing at first, especially when it is also multi-layered, but let us see if we can take this apart so that it makes sense.

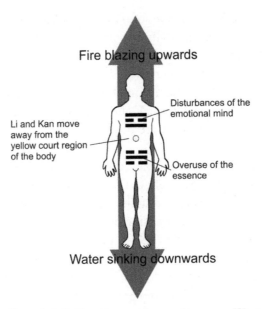

FIGURE 2.2: THE SEPARATION OF FIRE AND WATER

First, the copulation of the Dragon and the Tiger means different things on different levels. At the level of Jing (physicality) it can actually refer to sexual practices known as dual-cultivation practices. The male is the Dragon and the female is the Tiger. Specific tantric and energetic practices enable these two to combine their energies and so mix the Fire and Water essences with each other through physical union. This would be considered the lowest-level manifestation of Dragon and Tiger energies mixing and is generally only used within Daoist sects to form a foundation of good health within the physical level of the body. The second level of Dragon and Tiger mixing refers to the energies of the Liver and the Lungs, which can interact with each other at the Qi (energy body) level. This would take place within some forms of Qi Gong exercise. The third level can refer to the mixing of the spiritual energies of the pineal and pituitary glands, which will produce a fluid that moves through the body restoring health to many of the body's tissues. This is probably the least-used definition of the Dragon and Tiger terminology, to be honest, and it is mainly understood in this way within more esoteric Daoist sects concerned with attaining physical rather than spiritual immortality. The final (and most relevant to alchemical meditation practices) level is the meeting of the Yin line within the Li trigram with the Yang line within the Kan trigram. As this happens it is said that the positions of Dragon and Tiger have become reversed.

By subtracting the Yin line from the centre of the Li trigram we have found the Dragon. This can only be stirred by finding true stillness in the Heart-Mind through prolonged and diligent sitting practice. This will cause the Yin line to sink downwards, as 'to sink' is the true nature of Yin. In the early stages of the practice this will enable the Fire energy of the Heart to stabilise and stop rising, as it is now anchored into the body by the Yin 'Dragon' line. In the same way we must stimulate the Yang 'Tiger' line of the Kidneys to movement that will cause it to rise. This lifts the Kan 'Water' energy, preventing it from sinking as before. Now the ageing process is slowed and the early stages of alchemy have been entered into.

If we can do this for long enough and effectively enough we will cause the two centre lines to meet within the yellow court. This will result in the two lines 'copulating', which reverses the centre lines of Kan and Li. The result is the formation of the Qian (乾) and Kun (坤) trigrams, which are pure Yang ☰ and pure Yin ☷. Now Fire and Water will be gone and alchemically Heaven and Earth have been produced instead. This brings harmony to the body, which will in turn lead a practitioner towards true stillness, the emergence of the congenital nature (consciousness) and the dissolution of the acquired mind.

All of this is the precursor to ending the movement of the breath, mind and spirit to generate the three congenital treasures, the key ingredients that form the alchemical agent – the mystical elixir of Daoism.

3

WORMS
Damo Mitchell

It is an interesting characteristic of Daoism that models of human psychology, physical ailments and even subjects such as demonology are often interwoven with one another. For me it is one of the most fascinating facets of the tradition – the interwoven nature of the various realms of reality/manifestation and how this directly impacts upon many of their practices.

To give you a good example of these multifaceted teachings I would like to share with you the teachings of the San Chong (三蟲) or the 'three worms'. I was first introduced to the concept of the three worms, whilst staying in Beijing and studying at the white cloud temple over a decade ago. It was also a theory that I later came across in different schools and within classical written teachings. In each instance there was a slightly different take upon the theory of the three worms, though the underlying concepts were fundamentally always the same.

The three worms can be said to represent 'desires and wanting', 'attachments and regrets' and 'unconscious habits'. These are said to be the three key tricks that the mind plays upon itself in order to pull us away from a state of true consciousness. If we put these three aspects of mind into the context of a passing timeline we see the following: 'desires and wanting' are aspects of the mind that are, more often than not, applied to the future – things we want. 'Attachments and regrets' are those things that connect us to the past. It is our 'unconscious habits' that erode our personal willpower and keep us from being mindful of the present moment. These three facets are then embodied within the three worms as summarised in Table 3.1.

Table 3.1: The Three Worms

Name of worm	Location of worm	Facet of mind	Timeline
Peng Ju (彭琚)	The head	Desires	Future
Peng Jiao (彭瓚)	The sacrum	Habits	Present
Peng Zhi (彭矯)	The chest	Attachments	Past

In this instance the three worms are clearly aspects of the mind – three ways in which the mind is drawn away from the present moment. If we are drawn away from mindfulness – conscious awareness of the present – then the mind cannot grow still. Within alchemical Daoism this was the basis for the majority of human ailments. A lack of constancy or stillness within the spirit means that a person's essence and energy can become scattered or weakened. Though the worms are aspects of mind they are also located within specific areas of the body; this is where the crossover between the consciousness body and the physical body starts to take place.

The Peng Ju worm resides within the head; he has a relationship to the upper Dan Tien and our sense organs. As our mind races into the future and imagines things, people, places and events that cause us to desire them, it distorts the energy of the sense organs and disrupts the clarity of our mental faculties. It is also said that Peng Ju moves in and out of the body through a region towards the top of our neck around the occipital region known as the 'jade pillow' or Yu Zhen (玉枕).

The Peng Zhi worm resides within the chest and has an impact upon the region of the Heart that is also said to be the residence of human spirit. This worm relates to our attachments as well as regrets for events that have already come to pass. It is these attachments to the past that trap our mind and prevent us from evolving independently from past events. The Peng Zhi worm is said to move in and out of the body through the middle of the spine around a region known as the 'spirit path' or Shen Dao (神道).

The third and final worm is the Peng Jiao worm. This worm resides around the region of the sacrum. It has an impact upon the lower abdominal region as well as the lower Dan Tien. It relates to the development of habits. Habits are behavioural patterns that have developed to a point of being largely unconscious. These habits can on a simple level be small behavioural patterns that we automatically carry out without thinking or they can be more obviously destructive habits such as our addictions – 'drug habits' or 'drinking habits', for example. These habitual patterns cause us to lose our state of awareness and thus weaken our connection to the present moment. On top of this, habits are said to be in direct conflict with the development of will. It is only when our habits have been eroded that divine spiritual will is able to manifest within a person's being. Peng Jiao is said to move in and out of the body through the base of the sacrum.

It is clear to see from these descriptions that though the worms are primarily facets of mind, they are also seen as having physical locations within the body and are even personified to a certain degree, as they are able to move in and out of the body of their own accord. Within religious Daoism they take this even further and state that on certain days of the year the three worms ascend to Heaven during your sleep and report on your wicked deeds to the deities of judgement.

The location of the three worms also corresponds to three key locations upon the body that practitioners of alchemical meditation will be more than familiar with. These locations are known as three of the key 'clipping passes' – areas of difficulty for those involved in Daoist meditation. These locations are shown in Figure 3.1.

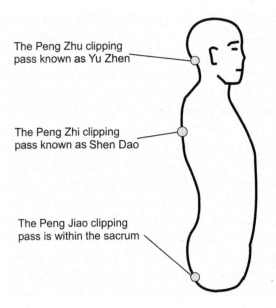

The Peng Zhu clipping
pass known as Yu Zhen

The Peng Zhi clipping
pass known as Shen Dao

The Peng Jiao clipping
pass is within the sacrum

FIGURE 3.1: THE THREE CLIPPING PASSES OF THE WORMS

They are considered difficult areas of the body to work through in your practice. One of the earliest practices within Daoist sitting meditation is the Xiao Zhou Tian (小周天) or 'small Heavenly orbit'. This is a circulation of information that moves up the back of the body and down the front through two of the largest meridians. Together these form an important orbit of Qi, which serves to transform and recycle energies back through the body during prolonged internal practice. When the energy begins to move up a person's back it is likely that it will become stuck in the three locations. Teachers have prescribed numerous methods to attempt to help practitioners overcome the challenge of the clipping passes.

One model of clearing the clipping passes that is pertinent to this chapter is the model of the three worms. If we use the example of the facets of mind related to the worms we can see that clearing the lower pass around the sacrum region would require the ending of habitual thought patterns and behaviours. To clear the second pass around the middle of the back a person would have to dissolve their attachments to the past, and to clear the upper clipping pass near the neck they would have to end their desires. As this happens, a person is drawn more into the present moment, their awareness of their own being increases and the mind grows increasingly still, and thus the rotation of the Xiao Zhou Tian should flow smoothly around its orbit.

The personification of the three worms goes further still within some schools of Daoism, and in these cases they give the worms form. They take the appearance of the three somewhat unusual-looking creatures shown in Figure 3.2.

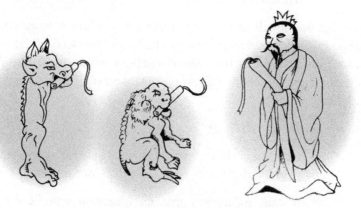

FIGURE 3.2: THE THREE WORMS' FORM

In the case of schools who adhere to this theory, the three worms are seen as demons or negative spirits who are the cause of many kinds of disease. People are thought to have been possessed by the negative traits of the worms if they are enabled to grow too strong. They grow as we feed them with our mind. Our desires feed Peng Ju, our habits feed Peng Jiao and our attachments feed Peng Zhi. If a person becomes 'overtaken' by any of the three worms, they can manifest some of the following symptoms:

- Peng Ju possession symptoms

  – A feeling of pressure in the head, chronic migraine-type headaches, weakened vision, poor hearing, unusual phantom smells and tastes, blotches and abnormalities upon the skin of the face, excessive amounts of mucus or spontaneous flowing of fluid from the eyes, bad breath.

- Peng Jiao possession symptoms

  – Digestive issues, weakness in the back and knees that limits mobility, weakness and cold in the lower abdomen due to damage to the lower Dan Tien, nocturnal emissions, excessive feelings of desire and lust, addictive behaviours.

- Peng Zhi possession symptoms

  – Pain and swelling in the chest and hypochondriac region of the body, shortness of breath, spasms in the body, an obsession with sensual pleasures, depression, suicidal tendencies.

As if this was not all grim enough there are even further worms within the body! Once again these 'beings' cross over into facets of the psyche as well as entities that have literal locations within the body. These worms are the Jiu Chong (九蟲) or 'nine worms' and they are named as follows:

- Fu Chong (伏蟲) or 'Trapping Worm'

  – Drains a person's essence and energy. Also said to feed off blood and generate toxicity in the bloodstream.

  – It was understood that an obsession with lower base desires would help to sustain this worm.

- Often treated in acupuncture through GV15 – Ya Men (啞門).

• Hui Chong (蛔蟲) or 'Roundworm'

  - Attacks the vital energy that motivates the movements of the Heart. This can result in low moods as well as a collapse of the Heart's energy and function.

  - This worm is nourished through prolonged periods of depression.

  - Often treated in acupuncture through GV14 – Da Zhui (大椎).

• Cun Bai Chong (寸白蟲) or 'Inch Long White Worm'

  - This worm eats into the digestive system, weakening the intestines, the Stomach and the Spleen.

  - Overly obsessive thought patterns were said to help this worm flourish within the body.

  - Often treated in acupuncture through GV13 – Tao Dao (陶道).

• Rou Chong (肉蟲) or 'Meat Worm'

  - The meat worm attacks the Liver, a person's muscles, their physical strength and the health of their spine and abdomen.

  - This worm takes hold of a person's body if they are harbouring large amounts of pent-up anger.

  - Often treated in acupuncture through GV11 – Shen Dao (神道).

• Fei Chong (肺蟲) or 'Lung Worm'

  - This worm causes unexplained conditions within the health of the Lungs. These conditions do not react to regular treatments.

  - This worm thrives within people suffering from long-term grief that they cannot move past.

- Often treated in acupuncture through GV4 – Ming Men (命門).

- Wei Chong (胃蟲) or 'Stomach Worm'

  - This worm eats its host's food, meaning that they always have a burning hunger that is never satisfied. They are also likely to become emaciated and weak.

  - This worm lives within those who have an overly active mind that is always scheming.

  - Often treated in acupuncture through GV5 – Xuan Shu (懸樞).

- Ge Chong (膈蟲) or 'Diaphragm Worm'

  - This worm weakens the energetic processes of the entire body, resulting in chronic fatigue-type symptoms.

  - Having a low spirit is said to strengthen this worm.

  - Often treated in acupuncture through GV3 – Yao Yang Guan (腰陽關).

- Chi Chong (赤蟲) or 'Crimson Worm'

  - This worm drains the Kidneys and causes ringing in the ear, pressure in the head and erratic thought processes.

  - This is the worm that lives off our fears and anxieties.

  - Often treated in acupuncture through the use of the lumbar Jia Ji (夾脊) points.

- Qiao Chong (蹺蟲) or 'Mobile Worm'

  - This worm moves around the body, especially under the skin. It causes unexplained itching, sores and rashes over the body that cannot easily be cured.

  - It is addictions to toxic behaviour that feed this worm.

  - Often treated in acupuncture through GV1 – Chang Qiang (長強).

This is where the multifaceted view of Daoism gets more interesting. The discussion of these nine worms clearly suggests that the ancient Chinese were actually talking about different types of parasitic worms that could physically and literally infest the body. They even went so far as to depict the nine parasitic worms as shown in Figure 3.3. As you can see, they are attractive little critters!

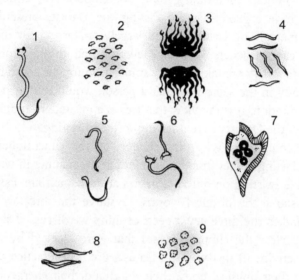

FIGURE 3.3: THE NINE PARASITIC WORMS OF DAOISM

Despite these worms being literal parasites that are a physical root for many kinds of disease, they are connected back to the three original worms that are as much metaphors for aspects of the human mind as they are types of spirit that reside within the body. As well as this, if we look at the meridian points classically indicated for the treatment of these worms we can see that once again they all sit along the key congenital meridian that runs along the length of the back. This is another indicator that treatment of the worms should be seen as a method of ensuring this key energetic pathway is open. Here we have the crossover between the physical, the spiritual and the psychological.

For another example of the way in which Daoist views and practices cross over into different realms we can look at one key suggested cure for 'worms' – Bi Gu (辟穀). Bi Gu means 'to abstain from grains' and refers to the act of fasting for periods of time. It was believed that the worms, both the nine parasitic worms and the three spiritual worms, sustained themselves on the grain that a person ate as well as negative emotions, and so periods of fasting was seen as the most effective manner to starve and kill them off.

Throughout history different spiritual cultures have acknowledged the importance of fasting and Daoism was no exception. The view of many sects of the tradition was that fasting was a required part of training to attain immortality. Many contemporary practitioners and scholars have argued that the fasting the Daoists prescribed was actually metaphorical and referred largely to 'fasting for the mind'. In many cases, teachers with this view will state that they are fasting when in fact they are taking away stimulation for the sense-functions of the body in the same way that a person would during periods of quiet meditation. It is my view that this is a misunderstanding and in actual fact the Daoists were referring to literal fasting.

The connection with the change of the practitioner's mind through fasting comes from understanding the manner in which they viewed life existing on different planes at the same time. Fasting was used to starve the physical worms, to starve the three worms that correspond to the three key aspects of mind we discussed above, and finally to clear the clipping passes that were blocked by the three worms' activity. In this way the Daoists used the practice of fasting to purify their physical body, their mind and their energetic system. In this aspect of their training the Daoists were not so different from many other traditions.

In presenting this information I did not wish to make people paranoid about the existence of spiritual and physical worms within their body! I did not want people to fear that the 'flesh worm' was currently eating its way through their intestines, and that is why they are held back in their practice. I merely wanted to present to you an example of the theory that came out of the Daoist tradition that pulled together models of the physical, the energetic, the spiritual and the psychological. Daoism is a colourful tradition and, as one of my alchemical teachers would tell me, 'feel free to let the worms eat your flesh, but don't let them eat your spirit!'... He always was a somewhat morbid fellow.

4

TALISMANIC FU
Damo Mitchell

A Daoist Fu (符) is a form of talismanic transmission. Originally, the term itself denoted a contract that existed between two people; it was taken from the practice of breaking a piece of jade or precious stone in half as a sign of mutual agreement. Both parties within an agreement would take half of the stone as a sign of their contract, their Fu, and by placing the two halves together could prove that said agreement existed.

Within the esoteric Daoist tradition, the Fu was taken out between the practitioner and the realm of Heaven, the abode of the immortals. This contract enabled the skilled Daoist practitioner to utilise the power of Dao (道) to establish a directed form of transmission into the talisman. This transmission would serve to change the quality of Qi within its immediate vicinity, which would then in turn generate a shift within the realm of manifestation. It can be thought of as placing a type of vibrational information into the symbol itself, which then sends this vibratory information out into the energy of the surrounding area. This information then causes a change within the 'flow of life' or Ming (命); this change could be to alter an area, an event or the Ming of a specific person. Figure 4.1 shows three examples of ancient Fu designs.

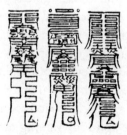

Figure 4.1: Fu Designs

Oftentimes Fu talismans were used as a way to ward off evil spirits, to increase the power of energy within a space or to tackle specific pathogenic imbalances within a person. In the case of the latter, the Fu was often either drawn on to the patient's body by a medically trained Daoist or burnt in pure water, which was then applied to the patient's body or drunk. When the Fu was placed into water in this manner it created Fu Shui (符水), which can be translated as meaning 'talismanic water'. If we think of how water can be absorbed into the human body, it is not so much a stretch of the imagination to see how energetically charged water could be useful for healing if generated in this manner.

In the case of magical Daoist traditions such as the Mao Shan (茅山) tradition, it was common for the practitioner to wear the talisman on their body for prolonged periods of time in order for the effects of the Fu to begin changing their own energetic flow. In the majority of these cases the Fu was seen as a spiritually binding contract between the Daoist and the deities that are such a large part of the more magical Daoist traditions. These Fu are generally placed upon the forehead of the arms of the Daoist or their abdominal region, as these areas correspond to the spirit of the practitioner, their ability to commune with the energetic environment and their personal power centre. Magical Fu such as these were highly prized, and it was understood that only the most powerful Daoist magician could create Fu of this magnitude. In many cases this level of Daoist practitioner was sought out by the emperors of China who would use their Fu to bind deities to their will in the hope of securing power in battle as well as in politics.

Within alchemical Daoism the Fu is often used to purify the area of practice as well as to help free the spirit from its bondage within the body. By placing the correctly formed Fu on certain areas of the body it was understood that the consciousness of the practitioner could begin to elevate itself above the lower realms of being. These Fu were generally placed upon the chest, the hands and the feet. Variations of this practice were also used to develop skills such as astral projection and remote viewing, though few Daoist schools in modern times still either recall or use these alchemical Fu practices.

In many parts of Asia, especially Hong Kong and parts of Malaysia, Fu can be bought in temples for varying amounts of money. In the majority of cases, these Fu are produced in batches and obviously contain little in the way of any power. Despite this, they sell to more traditional families who will place them around their house in order to improve the quality of their luck or protect them from evil spirits.

Only one who is able to enter into the correct meditative state can generate a working Fu. By taking the consciousness to a point of complete stillness they connect to the point at which Dao comes forth into the realm of conscious manifestation. Entering this state is challenging enough, but remaining in this state can be even more difficult. For many practitioners it is a challenge to get to this point, but even more difficult is retaining a certain degree of mental focus at the same time. The tendency for intermediate-level practitioners is for the entering into this state to come with a complete dissolving of the mind – a temporary state that results in a complete stilling of all conscious activity. With the potential for controlled focus lost, there is no way for any kind of vibrational information to be generated within this space. It is this information that must be generated by the practitioner if they wish to empower a Fu. The correct balance of stillness and focus is a high-level attainment.

For those who can attain this stage, the information held in their focus begins to manifest into various spiralling shapes, which look much like mandalas. With time and mental steadiness these mandalas begin to stabilise and form themselves into more constant isometric patterns, which essentially are the basis for the creation of Fu within the realm of manifestation. Essentially, the workings of the Fu generated in this manner come about because you are directly interacting with the substance of reality. Reality is, at its core, geometry. The geometric patterns that form in the mind's eye during meditation are the seeds of existence. When the interaction of focused will takes place then the geometric patterns form into an energetic pattern that can be perceived and then transferred into a physical format: a Fu. This will then have an effect upon the underlying geometric patterns of reality within the vicinity of the Fu. In this way the Qi of an area is changed.

The Fu are then drawn out according to the image perceived within the Daoist practitioner's mind and then they are empowered through the projection of energy into the symbol itself. Classically they were drawn on rice paper or thinly sliced bamboo, though they were also often carved into rock faces within sacred spots as well. In some parts of South East Asia I have come across practitioners, particularly within the fighting arts, who inscribe Fu onto semi-precious stones and insert them under the skin. As the skin grows back they are left with a spiritually charged 'lump' on their body, which they tend to use to generate more fighting prowess over their enemies.

For many, the idea of Fu and their usage can sound like complete fantasy or too far-fetched to even consider, but for many across Asia the power of the Fu is absolute.

For myself, I originally came from a point of viewing the Fu as outdated superstition, but as my comprehension of the power of vibratory information increased through alchemy training I began to understand how they could work. Now I have Fu around my living and training spaces as well several that are tattooed on my body. These symbols are there to adjust facets of my nature as well as to change aspects of my health. For me they are an adjunct to the Daoist internal process and an interesting aspect of an arcane tradition that hails back to its Shamanic roots. It is the nature of all societies to view those in the past as more 'primitive' and less 'advanced', when in actual fact it seems to me that the mindset was just very different.

The Fu are an element of this ancient way of thinking that has made its way through into modern times, though it is rarely understood any more, and it is interesting for me to see how the more time I spend around this tradition the more I embrace the Daoist approach to life. I no longer find a clash between the thinking behind the Fu and modern logic – something that I would never have thought would be the case when I was younger.

5

MASTERY OF FORM
(THE SIT)
Part 1
Damo Mitchell

Within the Daoist tradition there are various forms of sitting practice. In many cases these practices are all lumped under one category of 'Daoist meditation' and treated the same when in actual fact the different sects each have their own unique methods. Different terms are applied to different forms of sitting: terms such as Jing Zuo (靜坐), Zuo Wang (坐忘), Nei Dan Gong (內丹功) and many more. Some methods of sitting practice are distinctly Daoist in nature, whilst others have been influenced by other traditions, most commonly Chan (禪) Buddhism. Another distinction that exists between sitting methods is the degree to which they utilise the relationship between mind and body. Some methods almost exclusively place importance upon direct work with consciousness, whilst others work more evenly with the mind and its relationship to the body. In the case of these systems, the body is worked with through controlled use of the three internal treasures of Jing, Qi and Shen. Commonly translated as meaning essence, energy and spirit, work with these three aspects of human existence is designed to build a bridge between the denser realm of the physical form upwards into the more ethereal state of pure consciousness. Generally these forms of even mind/body sitting practices fall under the heading of internal alchemy within the Daoist tradition.

When beginning any form of sitting practice, but arguably it is most important within alchemical forms of practice, it is imperative that we learn how to sit. Now, to absolute beginners this can seem like an unusual statement. Surely sitting is something that comes naturally to almost all people and isn't it something that we spend a great deal of our time doing? The answer to this is that sitting down to engage in prolonged meditative training can actually be one of the most difficult things you have ever tried to do. For beginners, the very act of sitting still with little in the way of stimulation becomes the first hurdle as well as the reason why the majority of hopeful 'meditators' quit after a very short time. Despite these difficulties, learning to sit is very important if a person wishes to come to terms with the core of the Daoist tradition, and I always advise beginners within the arts to spend time learning this skill before they even bother trying to engage in the more complex aspects of alchemical practice.

Within Daoist alchemical meditation the most effective methodology for sitting practice is essentially to build a pyramid structure, with your hips spread open to form the base of the pyramid and the top of your head forming the tip of the pyramid. Within the centre of this pyramid we align the spine and associated energetic pathways so that they form a pole that runs from the centre of the pyramid's base up to its highest point. This structure should be relaxed throughout but with a gentle stretch applied to the soft tissues throughout the entire body. The reasons for this are based in the qualitative nature of Qi and the manner in which it moves.

Qi is a curious 'substance'. Generally, the translation of 'energy' is given to Qi, but this is somewhat inadequate as a definition. Qi is a wide term that can refer to a great many things within the Chinese language. With regards to alchemical meditation training Qi is something of a jargon term that does in actual fact refer to a kind of energetic 'substance' that flows through the body, but it goes deeper than this. This 'substance' is not a physical component of the body, and yet, to those who have experienced its activity, it feels very much like a fluid that moves through pathways within the body. It also has slightly magnetic and electrical properties, which, once again, can clearly be felt and experienced. These magnetic and electrical properties have a great effect upon the various fields that surround the whole of our body, the organs and even the cells themselves. When a Qi Gong master is seen manipulating the 'energy' of another person from a distance it is normally these magnetic and electrical fields that are being adjusted. A final component of the 'substance' of Qi is that it conveys information in the form of waves. This information is carried from our intent through the fields and flowing pathways of the body to govern the functional activities of the organs, tissues and every facet of human life. This information changes frequency in accordance with our thought patterns and emotions, and it is these changes that have a direct influence upon the quality of our Qi. From this explanation, we can see that it is difficult to pin down an exact definition of Qi within the body, as it is quite an abstract 'substance'. Despite this, we must develop some kind of a conceptual framework for what Qi is before we can hope to work with it. Of course, conceptual frameworks must remain flexible, and it is likely that they will change as a person develops in their practice. This adheres to the Daoist concept of non-definition, as absolute definition limits the potential for evolution.

The sitting posture for alchemical meditative practice is based around establishing a directional flow for the body's Qi so that it rises upwards towards the crown of the head. In this way it serves to nourish the energetic blueprint of the mind as well as to convert upwards in frequency to the realm of pure spirit. Over the years, I have travelled throughout Asia and studied various forms of Tantric (meaning 'works with energy') practice that aimed to raise energy upwards within the body. There are countless ways to achieve this aim, but I found many of these methods to be somewhat risky. This is because the majority of the methods I came across were based around forcefully lifting Qi upwards through the use of forceful breathing methods or strong mental focus. In many instances the energy of the base instinctual drive of sexual desire was used as a kind of mental 'fuel' for this lifting process – a method that has found its way into many Western schools of internal practice. In almost all of these methods there are many people who have damaged themselves both physically and emotionally, as they are using the wrong aspect of mind as well as a forced method. If you force something to take place, or use the lower aspects of mind, you go against what is natural, and thus there is always going to be an element of danger involved. Within Daoist alchemical sitting practice we never force anything nor use the mind to assist in the process. Instead we establish the 'pyramid' shape within the body and allow this structure to guide the movement of Qi according to a key rule of Qi flow: Qi will move to where there is space. In this way it can be thought of as being like water. Water will flow to fill any space, and Qi moves in much the same manner if it is left to move of its own accord. Within the pyramid shape of our sitting posture we have a feeling of fullness or density near the base of the body as well as establishing a feeling of lightness or emptiness towards the top of the pyramid. This takes place naturally and sets up the form of the alchemical practitioner as shown in Figure 5.1.

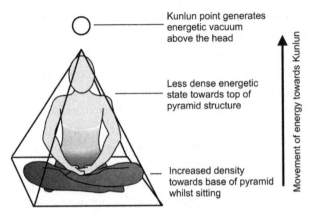

Kunlun point generates energetic vacuum above the head

Less dense energetic state towards top of pyramid structure

Increased density towards base of pyramid whilst sitting

Movement of energy towards Kunlun

FIGURE 5.1: THE PYRAMID STRUCTURE

The density or 'fullness' of the base of the pyramid is developed over time as the central axis of your body stretches upwards and the rest of your body mass relaxes downwards. The sinking of your body's weight begins to build a slight pressurisation against the base of the pyramid and in this way a region of dense energetic pressure builds up. The opposite of this is the fullness that is generated by the extension of the spine, neck and head. Directly above the top of the head is the Kunlun (崑崙) point. This is a spiralling energetic region of the auric field, which sits approximately 12 inches above a person's head. As the form of the pyramid becomes more stable over time the Kunlun point begins to expand outwards to generate a kind of energetic 'vacuum', which serves to draw Qi upwards through the practitioner's body. This is the emptiness that helps to move energy from the dense base of the pyramid upwards. It is through this point that many esoteric sects of alchemical Daoism state that Shen can return to original emptiness. When it opens there is a distinct feeling of expansion taking place above you whilst you are sat; some practitioners have reported a roaring sound that accompanies this stage of attainment, though I have never heard this sound myself. A clear reference to the opening of this point in Daoism is 'the opening of the flower above the crown'.

The full formation of the pyramid shape takes time; the body has to take shape, the separation of fullness and emptiness needs to develop and there has to be complete comfort whilst sat in this posture. At first you will have subtle sensations as a guide to show you how well you have achieved this, but in time you also find that you become aware of 'leakage' points. These are areas where your structure is not quite right. The result of this is that some of the Qi moving through your system moves out of the body into the surrounding environment. You will find that with ever so slight adjustments to the alignments of your soft tissues these 'leakage' points can be cleared and thus there is less in the way of energetic wastage during our practice.

An important theory that underpins Daoism is that every aspect of human existence has an energetic component. In the case of physical organs and tissues this is fairly simple to understand. This is the basis of Chinese medicine after all. What is a little more abstract to get to grips with at first is that this also applies to emotions and thought patterns. Within Daoism every thought, mental process and even character trait has an energetic component. Though our emotions do not take a literal physical form, they still manifest energetically. This becomes very important within alchemical training, as essentially we are attempting to shed unwanted emotions and biases that develop both reactive-type thinking and mental distortions – distortions that are preventing us from contacting the true consciousness that sits within the centre of our being. In many other forms of meditative training it is through observation of these aspects of mind that they begin to adjust. In the case of alchemical training, it is true that observation is still an important component of the practice, but we also use the theory of energetics to help us with the 'shedding' process. This happens as emotions can only adhere to our being if they have a certain energetic density to them. The more negative (from our point of perception) and traumatic an emotional experience, the denser it tends to be in nature. Fear, sadness and grief carry a lot more 'weight' to them than feelings of empathy and compassion. Those with even the slightest degree of internal self-awareness can feel this truth. How does the energy feel within the body during periods of depression? It generally feels as if it wants to sink and shrink in on itself. In the majority of cases this energetic quality then manifests through into a person's physical body, which then takes on a look of being contracted in on itself and heavy in nature. Alchemy essentially means to generate some kind of conversion – a change within the energetics of our being. In the case of these 'denser' emotions/thought patterns, the alchemical change is to make them 'lighter'. As we sit and observe the mind in our sitting posture, the correct development of the pyramid structure causes energetic frequencies to move upwards and decrease in density. This raises energy upwards towards the Kunlun point but also serves to dissolve much of the 'weight' sitting behind those parts of our psychological makeup that we need rid of. In this manner we are literally locating the energetic mechanics behind the process of letting go of stuck emotions and making these mechanics work for us. If the pyramid structure has not been formed, the form not been mastered, then these mechanics are not in place and so alchemical change takes place more slowly.

This is the practice I advise people to undertake when they wish to begin a regular sitting meditation practice. Before any clear alchemical methods are given they must first learn how to 'master the form' of sitting. For many this is a great challenge, but those who put in the time with this deceptively difficult posture will find that they have established a strong foundation upon which to build the rest of their training.

In the next chapter we will look at the second most difficult part of learning to sit – the nature of the human mind and its activity.

6

MASTERY OF FORM (THE MIND)

Part 2

Damo Mitchell

In the previous chapter we looked at the mechanics and practicalities of developing a sitting practice, in particular the posture itself. As stated previously, anybody seriously wishing to develop a regular sitting practice should spend a sensible length of time learning how to sit in this manner.

The next stage when learning to sit is simply to do just that. Before learning any complex alchemical methods, simply sit and see what your mind does. This process of observation will give you a chance to really encounter the movements of your psyche and see just how active the mind is. In our daily lives we are generally blissfully unaware of the constant churning of thoughts that our mind goes through. As soon as we sit still and do 'nothing' though, we are shown with acute detail just how incapable we are of silencing our acquired mind. For anybody who has ever tried to sit and 'meditate' this will be an obvious statement, but for newcomers to sitting practice it can be both surprising and immensely frustrating at the same time.

The process of engaging with your thoughts will generally take a practitioner through a series of stages that are pretty similar from person to person. The mind will usually cause us to have the following experiences.

THE MIND 'FIRING OFF'

The first thing we tend to encounter is the mind going through what I call its 'firing off' stage. This is the stage of our mind producing wave after wave of pointless nonsense. I call it nonsense as I am sure most internal practitioners will agree with me when I say that rarely does an overactive mind produce anything useful or profound when we first sit down to meditate. Do not expect deep philosophical insights; expect shopping lists, pop songs, thoughts concerning the last meal you ate and all the chores you still have to do that day. Along with this torrent of mental chatter come memories, random images, comedy voices, colours, shapes and countless other mental fabrications that really amount to little in the way of meaning.

For many this can be irritating, but in fact it is essential that you do not get annoyed with your own mind. Instead, observe, get used to what the mind is doing and try your best not to become too overly involved. The reason for this is that the acquired mind is much like an unruly child trying to get your attention. It will give you a series of thoughts, memories and images in an attempt to get your interest. As soon as any of these thoughts have your attention then a thought process is generated, a string of evolving mental processes that evolve out of that initial movement of mind. This is vitally important to understand for those wishing to start a meditation practice.

The reason why this string of thoughts develops is that the acquired mind is constantly working at building more 'layers' around itself. In this manner it is seeking a state of constant mental evolution through the process of accumulating more and more mentally fabricated information. The Daoist concept is that this process of accumulation is negative, as it keeps a person away from knowing what the true nature of their consciousness is. This is because these mental 'layers' serve as a kind of distorted lens that keeps us from viewing the authentic nature of our selves as well as our external reality. This is why the Daoists talk of the superior practitioner learning how to 'shed' their layers and thus find the truth within. The mind can only build these layers if we 'give it' our attention. The saying is that 'where the mind goes, energy flows', and this is certainly the case with regards to our mental activity. If our attention is given to any of these (generally nonsensical) thoughts then we fuel this thought with our own energy. The acquired mind now ascertains that we are 'interested' in what it has to say and so consequently it enables that individual thought to develop into an unfolding stream of mental activity for us to get caught up in. No doubt all of us who have engaged in sitting practice will have had this experience at some stage. What generally happens then is that we realise some time later that we have become distracted from what we were doing and so the thought process is broken. Once again we return to our task of simply observing the mind, and so the acquired mind gives up on that particular thought process and instead goes back to the stage of 'firing off' piece after piece of useless nonsense. In this way it is trying to tempt us with various pieces of enticing mental chatter to see if it can drag us back in again.

Now, it may sound as though this is pretty schizophrenic. I am discussing the mind as if it is in several parts and as if you have a few characters in your head competing for your attention. Of course, this is not the case – you have one single, unified consciousness. But this is not how it appears at first when you begin your practice. It is as if the mind fragments itself into parts in order to help you understand the process it is going through second by second each day.

THE ARGUMENT PHASE

After some time sitting you begin to become aware of this process taking place. The tempting nature of the acquired mind's activities becomes clear, and so instead you sit back and become more adept at avoiding those thought processes. Of course, every now and then you will make a slip-up and find yourself contemplating just why you chose that particular colour for the walls of your front room or some such nonsense, but on the whole you should find that it is easier to become somewhat detached from the movements of the acquired mind. In order to get to this stage you generally go through a phase I call the 'argument phase'. This is the stage in your sitting practice when you finally get fed up of the way your mind is behaving and start to argue with it. The conversation goes something like this:

Practitioner: Ah, now I feel like I am getting somewhere, it feels like my mind is getting quiet.

Practitioner's acquired mind: Yes, but what about those clothes you saw the other day in the shop?

Practitioner: Hmmm, that's true, I did like those shoes quite a lot... wait...what am I thinking, I am supposed to be practising meditation! Stop thinking about rubbish like this and get back to your practice.

In this way your awareness of engagement in mental chatter has generated a conscious response from the 'aware' aspect of your mind and so you find that you have begun to argue with yourself – truly schizophrenic behaviour!

This kind of argument should be avoided if possible, as any kind of mental disagreement like this creates a kind of psychological 'clash' within your mental space. This inner conflict generates a density of energy based upon your own irritation. When this happens you generate a type of mental 'stuck point', which fuels the layers of the acquired mind even more than a prolonged string of thought processes. The acquired aspect of your mind loves conflicts. Whether you end up in a position of feeling that you are 'right' or you just end up feeling bad about yourself, the result is the same. The acquired mind has had the chance to energise a part of its mental chatter, and more distortion is the result. This fascination that the acquired mind has with conflict is obviously then manifested in the outside world, explaining human beings' fascination with arguments, trivial disagreements and concepts such as 'right and wrong'. It is for this reason that almost all internal teachers will encourage you to simply observe what takes place in your mind with no judgement.

THE EMOTIONAL PHASE

The next stage a person enters after some time is what I call the 'emotional phase'. What is happening at this point in your practice is that you are starting to locate the emotional content that sits beneath each of your thought processes. Emotions are simply a form of energy, shifting in response to the movements of your mind. These energies carry with them information that is processed by your awareness to give you the experience of an emotion. This is recognised within Chinese medical thought, which is why therapies such as acupuncture can directly affect your emotional state. Surrounding each thought, mental process and acquired layer of your being is an emotional energy, meaning that every single thought that you have during your life has an underlying emotional quality to it. It is this underlying emotion that you start to have contact with during your sitting practice after some time. Obviously, there is a great deal of difference in scale between these emotionally charged events; a memory attached to a childhood trauma will have a very different level of emotional energy to a thought about your next shopping trip.

During your practice there will be an awareness of the movement of these emotional energies. In some cases these will be fleeting glimpses of an emotional feeling, whilst at other times it is possible for strong emotional reactions to take place. Essentially, the process for dealing with these rising emotions is the same as anything else that your mind generates. These are movements of mind, just the same as before. Once again, it is important to try and observe these reactions without becoming involved in them. If you give these reactions your 'attention' then you fuel them with energy, and in this manner you strengthen them. They become a repeating thought process like before and so more layers are built instead of being shed from the mind. In some cases practitioners can become too caught up in these emotional shifts, and in this case their practice actually becomes counter-productive. I was taught that becoming 'lost' on this path is a big trap for more introverted people who engage in Daoist sitting practice. These people generally get lost in their emotions and become either increasingly depressed or lost in a cycle of bliss-experiences that are as much a trap as a perceived negative emotional state. It is during this phase of working with your mind that many practitioners benefit from the advice of an experienced teacher. They can help to guide you through this minefield of a phase.

As before, if attention is given to these mental experiences then this serves to make them more 'dense' in nature. If we look at the previous chapter we can see that the aim of the practice is to 'lighten' substances within the mental body through awareness but non-involvement. When these experiences are 'lightened' they become more 'ethereal' and do one of two things: they are either alchemically transferred into spiritual energies that nourish the Shen or else they are shed from the body. Both of these are positive signs of progress and occurrences that can be directly felt after some time. When this happens it is like a 'sigh of relief' for your inner self.

BOREDOM AND THE PHANTOM ITCH

Not appearing in any particular order but still worth discussing are 'boredom' and the 'phantom itch'. Both are major hurdles to your sitting practice that need to be overcome. Boredom is a major factor in people quitting their training. For every diligent meditation practitioner who sits down each day to work on their sitting exercise there are countless people who have started, grown bored and quit. Boredom is a trick of the acquired mind that it plays on you when it really wishes to pull out all the stops in making you stop your practice. Why does it want you to stop? Quite simply the acquired mind thrives on stimulation. Stimulation generates mental engagement in a thought process, which in turn gives this process energy, and this serves to build more mental layers. These layers distort consciousness, and in this manner the acquired nature grows stronger. This is why so many classical texts instruct you to switch off your senses, sit in darkness, not seek stimulation and 'embrace the boring'. Unfortunately, the acquired aspect of your mind does not like the lack of stimulation that comes from sitting practice and so the experience of boredom is created. Boredom is your mind telling you to seek out stimulation to feed your acquired mind. In short, boredom is one of the biggest and most important hurdles for you to overcome if you ever really want to get anywhere with the internal arts, whether in meditation or within the martial arts and their countless repeated techniques. There is no secret that I have ever come across for ending boredom – students either go through it or they don't. Like anything else, it should be noted and observed, and do not become involved in it. I found that once the acquired mind realises that you will not give in to the boredom and stop what you are doing, the boredom fades. After this happens several times your patience goes up and boredom becomes something you rarely experience any more…or at least not when you are practising your arts!

A final 'trick' of the acquired mind worth mentioning is the appearance of the 'phantom itch'. In actual fact, the mind does not only produce random itches on the body but also aches, pains and other physical sensations that have no logical basis in any physical stimuli. The most common reaction seems to be a randomly appearing and almost torturously powerful itch that appears right on the end of your nose when you are trying to settle into your sitting practice. As with the feeling of boredom, it is simply another trick of the acquired mind attempting to get you to engage with it. As with boredom it should be acknowledged and then ignored. You will find that most of these sensations quickly fade once the acquired mind realises that you are not willing to give it the attention it requires to absorb your awareness. On the other hand, if you scratch the itch, in the majority of cases this starts a whole torrent of mental activity once more, as you have started the ball rolling on engaging with the mind.

So in conclusion, it is important that you note the various stages involved in establishing a regular sitting practice if you are new to the arts. First, a person should learn how to sit and then, second, they should learn to observe and not engage with the activity of the acquired mind. You could say that whilst doing this you are learning how to settle in and get comfortable with the idea of sitting meditation. I always advise beginners to simply sit and go through these processes when they begin to get involved in meditation, as it establishes a foundation that makes further practice much easier to progress into. From here, whatever system of meditation you are practising (for me and my students it is alchemy) will have its own methods and practices that you then need to start learning.

7

CHINESE FU DOGS
Damo Mitchell

If you have ever visited China or any Chinese temples you will have no doubt seen a pair of Fu Dogs guarding the entrance; in fact you may have even seen them outside of Chinese government buildings or large restaurants. Fu Dog is actually a modern term, with the original Chinese term actually being Shi (獅), which means a type of lion.

Shi guard entrances to Chinese temples in pairs; one represents Yin and the other Yang. The Yin Shi is female and the Yang Shi is male. Traditionally, the Yang Shi is supposed to be placed to the left of the entranceway if you are looking outwards, with the Yin Shi on the right. This represents the Yin and Yang balance of the body in harmony when looking outwards from the temple and in non-harmonious, protective mode when receiving visitors (potential threats).

Figure 7.1 shows two Shi or Fu dogs guarding the bottom of a staircase in a temple on Mount Wudang (武当).

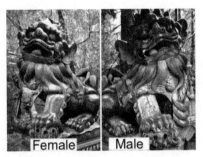
Female   Male

FIGURE 7.1: SHI OR FU DOGS

The two Shi shown in the example above are actually quite rare, as they depict the Shi slightly differently from the majority of examples you will see around China. The Yang Shi is stood upon a Xiu Qiu (繡球), which is a type of ball that features in many traditional forms of Chinese art. The Xiu Qiu is commonly hollow with several holes passing through it. Featured on its surface is a geometric pattern, which we commonly know as the 'flower of life' within the West. This pattern is formed from concentric circles, and you will find it appearing within architecture and artwork across all of the ancient traditions of the world. It is considered the sacred geometry of the cosmos – the mathematical representation of the formation of existence. Many alternative mathematicians have carried out considerable research into the geometric nature of existence, and many of these conclusions are contained within this shape. In the case of the Yang Shi it represents mastery of the macrocosmic nature of existence that sits within the centre of human consciousness. It is also the imagery that appears in front of the third eye when the golden flower has been accessed and a practitioner is able to perceive the geometric patterns that make up the fabric of reality. The holes in the ball represent the spaces that exist between the elements of this reality through which Qi weaves and winds its way.

The Yin Shi is often carved standing upon a baby Shi instead of a ball, although in the case of the example shown above she is standing upon a Xiu Qiu as well, whilst the baby Shi climb all over her. The baby Shi represent the formation of reality in a microcosmic way through the creation of a child. Some would argue that actually it represents the formation of the spiritual foetus within Nei Dan practice. In this way the two Shi balance each other – the Yin and the Yang; the nature of the creation of the microcosm and the formation of the macrocosm must be harnessed and brought together like two paired Shi in order to master one's self.

Often the Yang Shi, as in the case of the example shown here, contains a ball within its mouth. It is normally carved loosely enough to roll freely but it cannot be removed past his teeth. The ball is the alchemical pill or elixir formed through Nei Dan training. It can be passed upwards into the head of the practitioner, represented by the mouth of the Yang Shi. The Yin Shi does not contain one for a simple reason: she is classically carved with a closed mouth. The example above is a modern exception and both the Yin and Yang Shi have their mouths open.

The Yang Shi with an open mouth represents exhalation that is being used to stimulate the furnace of the lower Dan Tien. The Yin Shi classically has a closed mouth showing inhalation. The two must work evenly together in order to create inner harmony – inhalation and exhalation must be balanced. Within alchemy, respiration is everything; the spirit, the Qi and the consciousness move through the body according to the flows of our breath, and so mastery of breath is required at all stages of alchemical training.

The symbolic teachings of the Shi are valued aspects of the Daoist tradition. Standing at the entrance of most Chinese temples (and restaurants!) are guidelines on the overall philosophy of the practice of Nei Dan. One must control the breath, master the formation of the alchemical pill and bring together the powers of the macrocosm and the microcosm in order to attain spiritual elevation.

8

CLASSIC OF BREATH AND QI CONSOLIDATION

Damo Mitchell

Here is my translation of 'The Classic of Breath and Qi Consolidation'. This important Daoist classical poem discusses the relationship of Jing and Qi within the body as well as many facets of the 'microcosmic orbit' or 'small water wheel' of energetic circulation within the body. Despite being an important classic within Chinese alchemical circles, it is not so well known in the West.

It was planned as an appendix within my book *White Moon on the Mountain Peak: The Alchemical Firing Process of Nei Dan* but, alas, I ran out of time.

> In order to strengthen the Jing you should consolidate your Qi,
> To consolidate the Qi one must first bring the Jing to stillness,
> Use this method, master the Qi and the Yuan Jing will not disperse;
> If the Jing is consolidated, the Yuan Qi is no longer dispersed.
> The Yellow Court Classic[1] states:
> The consolidation of the Shen causes the Jing to still,
> In this way the old can be made young.
> The Jing that becomes Qi is transformed upwards,
> If the Qi is not made strong then the Jing is scattered.
> The Qi transforms to saliva and flows back downwards;
> If the Jing does not return to the source then the Qi is made imbalanced.
> It is like water being heated in a cauldron –
> If there is no Qi how will Qi be produced?

---

[1] The *Yellow Court Classic* is an ancient Daoist text that forms part of the Daoist canon known as the Daozang.

When Qi descends and is compressed we apply the warmth of the furnace and
*   it generates more Qi.*
If Qi rises without mental governance it disperses as emotions and is lost.
Though water flows downwards it is not shed;
If it flows upwards it is not lost.
As it flows upwards, water becomes Qi,
When Qi sinks it becomes water.
This forms the rotation of the water wheel.
The Yellow Court Classic states that this is the eternal path to immortality.
The result of the consolidated Jing and mastered Qi is evolution.
The vulgar people do not know the importance of mastery of Qi;
They do not practise this art and so they lose their Jing and Qi frivolously.
When Qi becomes Jing and is lost from the body it is useless.
When Jing becomes Qi and is shed from the chest it is wasted.
The Yellow Court Classic states that if you can consolidate the congenital,
*   mastery is yours.*
The elevation of spirit takes place within the workshop of your body.
Understand the art of transformation and contact Dao,
Dao is within the understanding of the body's natural cycles.
Through alchemical conversion returning to the source is certain.
Repeat the full cycle nine times and one will arrive at the stage of original being.

Below is a brief explanatory commentary on this classic. I have focused on key points with regards to alchemy from the point of view of a beginning-to-intermediate practitioner. The beauty of Daoist classics is that they are multi-layered in their meaning. You will often find that returning to them periodically yields very different understandings each time. These understandings will develop according to the level you have attained in your practice.

In order to strengthen the Jing you should consolidate your Qi,
To consolidate the Qi one must first bring the Jing to stillness,
Use this method, master the Qi and the Yuan Jing will not disperse;
If the Jing is consolidated, the Yuan Qi is no longer dispersed.

In this first section we are shown the cyclical relationship between Jing and Qi. Though Jing generates Qi, Jing also relies on Qi. Qi governs transformation, and so the conversion of Jing into fluids and developmental processes requires the existence of Qi. This Qi cannot exist without the generating action of Jing. The instructions here are to stop the 'scattering' of your Qi. This helps it to consolidate and thus help the Jing to convert in a more efficient manner. Qi is primarily scattered through emotions, and according to Daoism it is the interaction of your sense functions with the outside world that stimulates the mind towards emotional shifts. In short, consolidation of the Qi can generally only take place through learning to attain a state of inner stillness. This requires shutting off the senses through sitting meditation practice. Conversely, the Qi can only be consolidated if the Jing become still; this takes place through a combination of healthy living, adequate rest and moderation of sexual activity, as these all stir the Jing to movement. Sexual and base desires are a large factor in the 'movement' of the Jing and so great importance is given over to learning how to govern these sides of your nature. They were never denied but instead acknowledged for the natural and largely inconsequential mental factors that they are, and in this way a practitioner learns how not to be a slave to the desires of the Jing.

If you can achieve this then the Yuan Jing (元精), the original essence, will not disperse. The Yuan Jing is the true Jing that was given to you prior to your birth. It is one of the important substances in the generation of the alchemical pill. At the same time, as the Yuan Jing grows still, the Yuan Qi, original energy, will also consolidate to a state where it can be mentally contacted. The Yuan Qi is also required to start forming the alchemical pills – elixirs generated internally through mastery over the congenital substances. As a side note, the Yuan Qi is also sometimes known as Yuan Xi, original breath, within the classics. In essence Yuan Xi would be Yuan Qi when it is in motion.

> *The Yellow Court Classic states:*
> *The consolidation of the Shen causes the Jing to still,*
> *In this way the old can be made young.*

In the second section of the classic we are shown how the famed longevity aspects of Daoism come forth. Though they were never an original aim of Daoism they were a healthy by-product of the practices. If you manage to attain consolidation of the Jing and the Qi then the cyclical relationship between the two will begin to initiate consolidation of the Shen. This is human spirit, and when we can bring it to a certain state then the mind is stilled. This in turn generates more stillness within the Jing and thus the ageing process is slowed. We are being shown a clear sign of progress within this section of the classic.

The Jing that becomes Qi is transformed upwards,
If the Qi is not made strong then the Jing is scattered.

Through consolidation of the Jing, the Qi and the Shen we develop an efficient transformational process within the body. There is less wastage of the three substances of Jing, Qi and Shen through mental activity and inefficient internal activity. The result is that the Qi begins to rise upwards within the body as an advanced aspect of the microcosmic orbit that is a well-known part of Daoist Qi Gong practices as well as alchemy. In essence, this circulation takes place on many levels, with the most basic being the circulation of acquired Qi through the Du and the Ren meridians. At higher stages this circulation takes place as the Jing to Qi conversion is heightened, resulting in a flow of Qi through the deeper channels of the back and spine.

Here there is also a brief warning of possible problems at this stage. The Qi must be strong and healthy when you reach this stage in your practice. If it is not then the Jing will start to move once more. Consolidation is lost and the foundation of your work is weakened. A clear sign that practitioners experience is when they try to initiate the rising of the Qi and they are suddenly overwhelmed by sexual desires and erotic fantasies. This is because the Jing has become hyperactive as the Qi is not strong enough to support its stillness. If this happens over a long period of time then you run the risk of developing an imbalance known as 'poison Fire affects the Heart'. This is referring to a rising of impure Qi driven by sexual desire. Over time this starts to pervert the emotional standpoint of the Heart-centre; sexual deviances and fetish-like behaviours can manifest. In extreme cases it has been known that paedophilic tendencies can occur, though in many cases it simply turns into a supercharged sex drive. In the case of this starting to happen you should return to your foundation practices and return to this level of training when you have fully established a firm footing in the basics of work with Jing, Qi and Shen.

The Qi transforms to saliva and flows back downwards;
If the Jing does not return to the source then the Qi is made imbalanced.

When the true Qi of the microcosmic orbit reaches the top of its cycle it starts to convert into fluids. These fluids manifest as large amounts of saliva, which contain vital essences. They should be swallowed down with the gentle intention of them reaching the lower Dan Tien. When this happens the vital substances complete their internal orbit. The

Jing that had become Qi becomes saliva and then back to Jing. This is required if there is to be no leakage of Jing. It is needed back at the start of the orbit in order to keep generating Jing. This is vitally important to understand. We always wish for a transformational cycle that works to convert from Jing upwards and then back down into Jing. If we do not 'recycle' then imbalance in the Qi is the result and so the root of problems in our practice is established.

It is like water being heated in a cauldron –
If there is no Qi how will Qi be produced?

This is a direct reference to the conversion of Jing to Qi within the Ding, the 'cauldron' at the centre of the lower Dan Tien. The Jing is often represented metaphorically with the element of water, which is in part due to its classification as a very Yin substance whilst at the same time being a reference to the important role that Jing has in the creation of various body fluids. There is heat involved because as Jing transforms into Qi it generates an expansion inside the lower abdomen. The result of this is a clear feeling of inner warmth as well as, commonly, a sensation of something bubbling in the belly, much like something being brought to boiling point within a cauldron.

We are also, once again, reminded of the importance of recycling the Qi as there must be an energetic catalyst for everything that takes place. Qi is the great transformer, the bringer of change, and so its presence is required for anything to take place within our body or indeed the entire cosmos.

When Qi descends and is compressed we apply the warmth of the furnace and
it generates more Qi.

The 'compression' being discussed here is the retraction of the lower abdominal muscles as well as the raising of the perineum (some schools state that it is the anus rather than the perineum, though in practice I find little difference). This contraction of the lower abdominal region causes the Qi to be compressed within the Ding along with the Jing. This is what serves to 'cook' the substances and thus begin the alchemical process of change inherent within Nei Dan. Detailed instruction on this process is generally required in order to progress safely and effectively. I would advise seeking out a teacher for this in order to receive first-hand instruction, but if you feel you would like to read about the practice then you can refer to my book *White*

Moon on the Mountain Peak: The Alchemical Firing Process of Nei Dan. In this book I cover the foundations of alchemy, including this process, in great detail.

> *If Qi rises without mental governance it disperses as emotions and is lost.*

I am not sure whether it is disrespectful to criticise a classical text but I am about to. If there are any immortal spirits becoming angry at me right now, I am terribly sorry!

I have often felt that this line from the classic is a little misleading, as it may sound like it means we need to use the mind to govern the Qi. This misunderstanding has dictated the methods of many contemporary schools that prescribe using the intention to forcibly raise the Qi upwards within their body. This is often used in conjunction with focusing upon certain meridian points along the Du and the Ren circulation in an effort to directly generate the microcosmic orbit. The result of this kind of practice is generally that a strong tangible sensation of Qi movement can be felt but it is then weaker when you are no longer focusing upon directing the movement yourself. The use of the intention also disturbs the Jing, which is no longer still, and so a weak foundation is built for further development. With the foundation weakened the Qi then disperses and students may experience a range of results, which can include heightened emotional swings, feelings of anger, depression or, in a small percentage, more severe reactions.

The true circulation must be generated through working with the furnace and the cauldron and building a systematic conversion within the Jing, Qi and Shen as they stabilise. This is the method outlined within this text.

The 'mental governance' it is referring to is the 'governance of your own mental state', as in: keep your mind still and focused upon what you are doing. Do not become distracted and aim for a gentle but firm meditative state of awareness throughout the entire process. If the mind moves through a lack of governance then Qi becomes emotion and thus it is dispersed.

> *Though water flows downwards it is not shed;*
> *If it flows upwards it is not lost.*
> *As it flows upwards, water becomes Qi,*
> *When Qi sinks it becomes water.*
> *This forms the rotation of the water wheel.*

This section is essentially a summary of what is taking place if you practise correctly. It reminds us that 'recycling' the Jing through the body as more refined substances and then back again is the key to the water wheel, another term for the microcosmic orbit. In this way our inner environment is directly matching the water-cycle of the external world.

The Yellow Court Classic states that this is the eternal path to immortality.

A rather grand claim, but in theory this can lead you towards the highest levels of attainment within the Daoist tradition.

The result of the consolidated Jing and mastered Qi is evolution.

Evolution is of prime importance to Daoists. They recognise that there is a natural process of transformation taking place within us all of the time. This process is directed by the Jing and then adjusted by the emotional content of Qi, combined with the awareness of Shen. We will not stop the process of transformation taking place on a daily basis within us, but we can learn to master its energetic mechanisms and gently direct it in a more healthy direction. This is the Daoist path of spiritual evolution.

The vulgar people do not know the importance of mastery of Qi;
They do not practise this art and so they lose their Jing and Qi frivolously.
When Qi becomes Jing and is lost from the body it is useless.
When Jing becomes Qi and is shed from the chest it is wasted.

The 'vulgar people' is both a somewhat politically incorrect term for those people in the world who do not practise Daoism and a metaphorical term for the sense functions, which are thought of as having their own form of consciousness. This sense-consciousness is linked to the generation of emotional responses. In this way the text is telling us that our senses and our emotions are no aid for the oath to governing our Qi efficiently.

Our Jing and Qi should not be shed from the body (Qi is lost through the chest as emotions from the middle Dan Tien) any more than they have to, as once they are gone they are useless to us.

The Yellow Court Classic states that if you can consolidate the congenital,
mastery is yours.

It is common within classical spiritual texts to refer back to even older spiritual texts. In this way the writer is humbly showing that their knowledge came from those before them and that they deserve no credit for any achievements. It also helps to lend credibility to the text's teachings.

The elevation of spirit takes place within the workshop of your body.

Your body is your workshop. The external alchemist had his alchemy room, and the internal alchemist has their body. The workshop must be well maintained in order for good results to take place. We should maintain our physical health and well-being to the best of our abilities if we are going to make our 'workshop' an effective place to carry out our work.

Understand the art of transformation and contact Dao,
Dao is within the understanding of the body's natural cycles.

Dao is the indefinable source of all existence as well as the underlying truth that permeates throughout all of existence. To define Dao is impossible with either words or the intellectual mind; it can only be experienced. This experience can only come through contacting these natural transformational cycles within our energetic system and working with them to make them more efficient. Then we observe and maintain our practice in order to move deeper into Daoism.

Through alchemical conversion returning to the source is certain.

If you practise this method and master it then your spirit will be led back to the source, the original state of true being that Daoists seek. In contrast to many other traditions, Daoism did not believe that human spirit had to be taken to a higher state. Instead, the evolution process they discuss actually sheds the distortions that prevent us from operating according to the original state of being that sits within each of us, the source of all awareness that can directly contact Dao.

Repeat the full cycle nine times and one will arrive at the stage of original being.

Many practitioners mistakenly believe that they must circulate these energies a literal nine times in order to master the method. This is really not the case. Numbers are often used metaphorically within Daoism (as with many other esoteric traditions) and we must understand what this number means. Nine is the number of Heaven. Three is the first Yang number (Yang is odd) within Daoism, as the number one is considered a 'whole' number representing full union. Two is Yin as it is even, and so three is the lowest Yang number. Within Daoist symbolism we have the Gua or sacred symbol of Heaven as shown in Figure 8.1. This symbol is made up of three solid Yang lines.

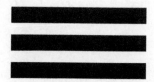

FIGURE 8.1: THE HEAVEN GUA

Each line is Yang and so numerically is represented by the number three. There are three of these lines, and so three multiplied by three equals nine. Thus nine is the number of Heaven.

Essentially, by utilising the number nine, the classical text is showing us that we must follow the way of Heaven. Heaven is eternal (as stated in the *Dao De Jing* (德道经)) and unmoving. In this manner we must sit beneath the teachings of Heaven and be patient and persevering in our efforts. Alchemy takes time, and we must be prepared to dedicate much time and effort to our training if we are to attain the Gong Fu or alchemy through the method outlined here.

9

MING MEN
Damo Mitchell

A fascinating aspect of Chinese medicine is its rich connection to the ancient beliefs of the Chinese people. It is part of the beauty of the art that the patient is seen in relation to his or her path through life and destiny as much as with regards to what is directly ailing them.

Sadly, in modern times this side of the art is rarely studied and instead it has been turned into a mechanical practice where the underlying concepts of Xing (性) (nature), Ming (命) (destiny) and De (德) (virtue) are ignored in favour of depersonalised point prescriptions. It was a key facet of the Daoist approach to medicine that each patient was looked at in conjunction with each of the aforementioned three elements of their existence. The relationship to and the manifestation of Xing and Ming as viewed through the lens of the distorted spirit was required in order to understand the larger picture of what was taking place for the patient. Originally, at its most profound levels, a treatment with Chinese medicine was supposed to aim towards realigning a person with their spiritual path as well as simply helping them with an ailment such as back pain. In an age where personal cultivation is all but ignored and material gains are the key measure of a person's success in life, it is no wonder that much of the beauty of the art of Chinese medicine has been lost.

One such aspect of the art is the use of the term 'Men' or 'gateway'. Several points upon the meridian system have the word 'Men' within their title – undoubtedly the most well known of these is the fourth point upon the governing meridian, which is known as Ming Men (命门) or 'the gateway to a person's Ming'. Figure 9.1 shows the location of this meridian point.

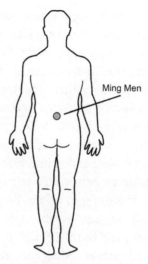

Ming Men

FIGURE 9.1: MING MEN

To the Daoists, a gateway was used as a metaphorical reference to a point that exists between the Xian Tian (先天) (congenital) and the Hou Tian (後天) (the acquired). Within the nature of energetics these two can be thought of as the difference between the potential for something to manifest and its actual manifestation. In the case of Ming Men it is referring primarily to the manifestation of the acquired Jing (essence) from the stillness of the Yuan Jing (original undifferentiated essence). This is the stage whereby human life manifests from its prior state of pure consciousness through into the realm of physical creation. This can be thought of as the initial point whereby human life is split away from the unified state of Dao into the dual state of existence we generally understand through a study of the comparative terms of Yin and Yang.

Most practitioners of Chinese medicine will understand that the Ming Men meridian point has a strong connection to a person's Jing, as well as the poles of Yin and Yang through the body. In many cases it will also be connected to the health of the Kidneys and the lower spine, though these physical aspects of the body exist at the absolute fringe of the range of potential manifestations of Jing; in short they are the branches and not the root.

What this means is that a skilled practitioner is able to utilise Ming Men as a point to be stimulated/worked with in conjunction with accessing the patient's spirit in order to contact the gateway of their existence. Balance can be brought into a patient's Ming – an element of destiny that dictates a person's very journey through life.

It is an important concept within Daoism that each person contains within them the un-actualised seed of Ming. This is like a set of blueprints for the path that a person will take through their life, including the inherent strengths and weaknesses that they will encounter over the course of their daily lives. In some traditions the seeds of Karma are also an aspect of a person's Ming, though of course these are concepts that were added into Daoism from other traditions at a later stage in its development. The strength of a person's Ming is, in part, dictated by the strength of the Jing gifted to them through their family line and in part by the nature and situation of their conception, pregnancy and birth. Though there is a range of strengths and weaknesses that a person's Ming may include, each of us has the potential for profound states of spiritual comprehension if only we are able to understand our Ming and learn how to move within its flow. When we can do this then the art of Wu Wei (無為) (non-governing) spontaneously manifests within us and, in the case of medicine, a person's Shen will vibrantly shine forth.

Sadly, self-expression and freedom are aspects of life that so often elude us due to restrictive pressures placed upon us. Consequently, many people move out of synch with their Ming. As this happens, imbalance is created and the poles of Yin and Yang within the body begin to move out of a state of harmony. This is a key source for the development of disease and an important facet to take into consideration for the sincere practitioner of Chinese medicine. The diagnostic process that looks at these aspects of human existence takes place through study of the relationship of the person's spirits, as these are conscious manifestations of a person's state of relationship with the wider sphere of Heaven.

The use of Ming Men gives a practitioner a point through which to access the original space within the energy body that lies at the source of a person's Ming. As it is treated, the barrier between the potential for Ming connection and manifestation of a person's life is bridged and this gives the therapist an opportunity to bring a person back in line with a deeper sense of self-purpose. The stages beyond this involve working with a person's Ming via the spirits, as these are required to move into harmony with each other, and the cycles of Yin and Yang, in order for flow along the line of destiny to continue in a healthy manner.

Ming Men is a powerful and transformative point, which should be treated with respect due to its potential strength. For the practitioner who wishes to understand the spiritual aspects of Chinese medicine, learning how to read the symbolism of Chinese medical terminology can be as complex as understanding a Daoist alchemical text, but the effort is worth it. All of the information is already there in front of us – we just need to move deeper into a study of the ancient teachings to bring back the potential of this ancient art form.

Alternatively, if you prefer acupuncture as a mechanical form of pain relief, save yourself all the complex study; just use this point for helping alleviate backache! This is a real shame though, as Chinese medicine has been through several periods of persecution in Chinese history. In each of these phases of its development it lost more of its potency and spiritual depth. We now live in a time where no matter how many pressures are upon us, there are little to no restrictions upon how we apply the teachings of Chinese medicine as therapists. More and more people are becoming interested in receiving treatment for deeper aspects of their being, and the information is right there in front of us if we can only understand the original philosophy. I feel that more therapists should use the freedom of expression they have and explore the deeper ethos of their system; in this way I hope it can be restored to a powerful and deep system of healing as it once was.

10

BECOMING CHRIST
Damo Mitchell

It is an interesting aspect of human nature that we often wish to seek out some kind of higher purpose. This may be through the practice of an internal art such as Qi Gong or Yoga, through study of self-help books written by modern Gurus or through aligning ourselves with one of the many religions that exist, across the world. It seems that ordinary life, though temporarily pleasing in many ways, simply is not enough for a great many people who wish to find out what the 'real' meaning of life is. Perhaps we could argue that the passion many people have for turning to science for answers is a manifestation of the same need. The new 'religion of science' is now probing the cosmos for answers as to what exactly makes us exist, and its followers are equally as passionate as any church-goer.

It is interesting for me to see how these different paths unfold for people across the world. In the last decade I have travelled through 30 or more countries on several different continents. In each of these places a different 'system' is giving people a chance to search for the answers they are looking for in a different way. I have spent time in Christian countries, Buddhist countries, Muslim countries, Hindu countries and places where scientific reason rules. In each of these places I had the chance to see how these systems guided people and how absolutely sure the people there were that they alone had the 'right' answers. All other systems were completely wrong; even if they do not say it aloud for political correctness reasons, I am pretty sure that many deeply religious people feel it deep inside. It is a strange trait of human beings that this concept of being 'right' gives us great comfort, as it lifts us above our fellow homo sapiens in some way. Strangely, many people seem to overlook the fact that their religion is largely a direct result of the geographical place of their birth more than a sought-out profound truth. Sadly, many will then shed blood in defence of this conceptual framework that was given to them without ever really considering that they would most likely have been equally defensive of the 'other' religion if they had been born elsewhere.

In many of the countries I have been to I have seen how problems between the different religions there have led to violence. Churches fight against mosques, and blood has run as each faction's god seems to have told their followers to kill the other god's followers. On a worldwide scale this has obviously been going on for centuries and different gods seem to be telling their followers to attack different groups on a whim, including, at different times, non-believers, other religions, witches, homosexuals, other races and potential terrorists. What strange beings gods are that they order people to do such things when they have the power, apparently, to wipe us out with a great flood whenever they want to anyway.

To me a religion is simply a spiritual system. It is a path that was originally developed to help people grow. It is a form of Nei Gong to me with a whole load of 'stuff' attached to it. If we actually look at the lives of people like Buddha or Jesus it is clear to see that they were highly advanced internal practitioners. Through deep insight and diligent practice they had reached such a level of divine awareness that they naturally had a great effect upon those around them. Let us be clear though, Buddha was not a Buddhist and Jesus was not a Christian; these concepts did not exist at that time. These were individuals who stepped out of conventional religious thought during that period and developed a way to teach people to advance themselves through self-analysis and compassion. Some might argue that Buddhism is not a religion, but I would say that it is, as it has monks, priests and a hierarchical structure. As soon as any spiritual group develops these and reaches any great size it has become a religion. I believe that, politically, Buddhism tries to state that it is a philosophy rather than a religion so that it can distance itself from the atrocities committed on a daily basis worldwide by the other religions – a stance I find completely understandable. The same has happened to Daoism. Now, I don't actually consider myself a Daoist, I am simply Damo, but I happen to find the teachings and methods of Daoism the most effective for what I am trying to do. Daoism in modern times is also a religion with monks and hierarchies in the same way as Buddhism. If I were to claim to be Daoist, I would no doubt have to accept that I was following the Daoist religion.

Please understand what I am saying though – this is not an attack on religion itself; there is nothing wrong with any religions at their heart if we look at the original teachings that underpin them. To be honest they are all pretty similar; it is only once people add layer after layer of their own interpretation and developed hierarchies that they become kind of nonsensical. I have a sneaky feeling that if Jesus, Buddha, Mohammed and various other high-level internal adepts sat down and had a chat they would get on swimmingly. I also suspect they would be rather horrified at what has gone on in their name.

What took place was that the external worship and ritual became more important than the original message of oneness and compassion, and straightaway problems developed. Now the 'tail was wagging the dog' so to speak, and their function was forgotten. It is my strong belief that anybody can find the spiritual answers they seek through any system and any religion, but they must understand when to step away from convention as the founders of these religions did themselves in the first place. The system can only take you so far before you get lost in the mire of ritual; they should be treated as methods that can open the door for you but then, once the fundamentals have been learnt, a person must seek their own answers. The problem is that people following religions are trying to be good Christians, Buddhists, Hindus, Daoists, etc. What are they doing? These people should be striving to be Christ, Buddha, Krishna or Laozi (老子)! These were people on earth who attained spiritual liberation from the constructs of their worldly form through their practices. They did not have grand churches, temples or golden statues of themselves to worship. They had a simple method of personal liberation that they developed and followed in order to attain the states of consciousness that they did. Existing religions were not their way, although they were all pointed in the right direction by the religions existing around them at that time.

What is wrong with aiming to be Christ or Buddha? By all accounts they were pretty decent people. It seems to me that the systems that developed around them after their death have only served to divide people from those states by adding lots of unnecessary 'stuff' – 'stuff' that causes division and strife between groups.

Daoism has certainly fallen foul of this. In the first instance there was a person (or group) who discussed a way in which to elevate the consciousness through simple living, non-conventional thought and meditation. As time went on, more and more complexity developed from this and now in Daoism there are gods, temples, monks, ritual, etc. Daoism fell into the same trap as Christianity, Buddhism, Hinduism, etc. People are lost in the rituals once more and cannot find their way to the true message. The rituals can serve a purpose at the beginning. That is all. Once there is no need for them they should be dropped and the essence of the system sought out. It should be sought out through simplicity. Even science is no different. Scientific thought can lead you so far, but the great discoveries of science were all made by those who dropped conventional thought and stepped outside of the system. First labelled as 'crackpots', they became scientific geniuses, the prophets of the science of religion.

So why don't people step away from external ritual into the simplicity of their systems? I think that there are several reasons. First, it is comforting to stay within the rituals; to move away from them is to enter a land of uncertainty and lose the 'comfort blanket' of external belief. Second, those in charge often have a vested interest in keeping you within the rituals because this means that those leading the rituals are still required; the middleman who allows you to communicate with your god through them is still in control. Third, I believe that it is because many religious people don't actually have total faith in their own religion anyway. If people actually believed deep down inside of themselves with no doubt whatsoever that their religious doctrine was true then they would not need the rituals; they would find their own way to god. If people fully believed their own religion to be real at their core they would not need to kill others to prove it. If you tell me that the sky is green, I will not kill you. I will not become angry with you, as I have no doubt that the sky is not green. You can keep saying it until you are blue in the face but it will not bother me; I will simply think you are crazy. Clearly, you are not speaking the truth. But, if somebody tells a religious extremist that their god is not real, then there is a good chance that they will become defensive and angry. Why is this? Are they not as certain of their belief as the sky is blue? Well, I believe that they have doubt. You will usually find that people expend the most energy defending something that they are actually unsure of themselves. You have touched upon that little glimmer of doubt that sits right there within them that prevents them from knowing wholeheartedly that they are actually 100 per cent correct.

So why the doubt? In my opinion it is because of ritual trimmings. Many people engaging with religions are so lost in the ritualistic actions that are a part of their system that they have never actually experienced a connection to god or a higher purpose. The ritual has kept them away from actually going inside the deep, quiet place many religions strive to lead you towards, as this is where your god will be found. In this profound emptiness, you have the opportunity to experience the very nature of existence. Once this experience has been had, there is no doubt – you have touched upon the seed of creation, the spark of 'god' that exists within your soul. Those few who have reached this stage are often said to have been 'spoken to by god' and deemed saints. They have taken the first step towards becoming Christ, Buddha or any of the other spiritual prophets of the ancient times. When this happens there is no need for ritual, external religious behaviour, visits to churches to confess your sins or anything else like this. You have found your own way to spiritual growth, a way that is deeply personal to you and yet at the same time universal across all colours, creeds and indeed religions.

To me, this is one of the greatest meanings hidden within the instruction of 'learn and then forget' attributed to Laozi. Find your way through convention and then be prepared to step out of it when it is no longer needed, for the only way is no way.

11

EXCITEMENT KILLER
Damo Mitchell

A side effect of prolonged training in the internal martial arts rarely discussed is the adjustment of what I call your 'excitement threshold'. This is the degree to which you can be stimulated by external events before reacting by becoming excited. The more you train in the internal arts, the greater this threshold becomes and the higher the level of stimuli required before you feel the pulse of energy, warmth and adrenal flow that previously came much more easily.

A while back my wife (Roni Edlund) and I had arrived in the town of Surat Thani on the Southern mainland of Thailand. We were on a short stopover before we headed into another part of Asia for training under a Taijiquan (太極拳) master. When we got to Surat Thani we caught a taxi, which was basically a pick-up truck. Sat in the back, it was a nice trip through the busy streets in the open air on our way to our hotel on the other side of town. About 20 minutes into our trip we were forced to stop due to protesters filling the roads; political upheaval is common in South East Asia, though on this occasion we had thought that the protests were confined to Bangkok. A crowd of Thai protesters marched past waving flags and banners as we sat in the traffic. Initially the feeling was more akin to a festival than a political protest, but suddenly the mood changed completely as shots started ringing out; somebody was shooting into the crowds and bullets were ringing off the cars on the street that our pick-up truck taxi was on.

The road cleared very quickly as pedestrians ran for cover and mopeds sped past with their riders ducked low behind the handlebars. Our taxi was not so quick to vacate the area, due to it being a large vehicle, but it too headed out of the street as quickly as possible.

As I heard the shots I turned to Roni and got her to duck down in the truck next to the bags and then I did the same. The one thing that struck me from all of this was that I did not feel any panic, stress or excitement whatsoever. The street had quickly erupted into chaos but it did not even register with me emotionally.

This experience parallels previous events that had taken place over the last few years. One previous winter I was repairing the roof of our Daoist shrine in Sweden. I was up on the roof in the snow with my student Tom. It was definitely not the wisest time of year to be working on a roof, but neither of us had really considered this at the time! I grabbed hold of the chimney to swing around to the other side of the roof from where I was working and a large part of the chimney came away in my hand. I fell with some bricks backwards onto the roof and landed with my head hanging over the edge of the building. In previous years this would have been one of those times when the heart 'skips a beat' and adrenalin would have kicked in. Instead I just picked myself up and carried on working; I was very calm and nonchalant about the whole thing. I had not really registered the accident emotionally and neither had my adrenals.

When I think back to studying the external martial arts, I would always finish a class feeling very excited. The nature of the training had fired me up and it would often be difficult to sleep directly afterwards if I was training at night. This is never the case for the internal arts, even if training Xingyiquan (形意拳) or Baguazhang (八卦掌), which are also martial systems that can often be practised at relatively fast speeds.

I believe what is happening is that when you move through sequences such as Taijiquan forms and engage in extensive training of Tui Shou (推手) (pushing hands) you are gradually releasing excitement-generating chemicals into the body to a very small degree. Energetically, you are causing excitement of the body's Qi but at a much smaller level than in the external arts. What happens as you do this is that you give your body and mind time to 'normalise' this state. As it gets used to these small amounts of energetic and chemical releases it stops registering them. Over time, the increased pressure of pushing hands and further combat drills 'ups' this amount of excitement and again your body and mind get used to them, meaning that it does not change your state of being. This process of increasing stimulation and then normalising it carries on throughout your training until you are able to move very quickly and forcefully or even fight without registering any bodily changes inside. I believe (though it is only my own opinion from personal experience) that this is one aspect of 'centring the mind' in the martial arts that brings about large degrees of calmness even under pressure. Obviously, further centring takes place on a more spiritual level, but I believe that too often the chemical changes are underplayed.

This of course transfers across into your everyday life, creating the large 'excitement threshold' that I gave examples of above.

The positive side of this is that you are able to think and act clearly no matter what the circumstances. Even under great stress you are able to function from a centred point of stillness without your thought patterns being compromised by your own state of inner excitement. This helps with protecting the Kidneys' essence, which is drained through stress, and so this in turn guards your physical and mental well-being. If adrenalin and excitement are not present in your body then you can maintain a steady control on your own internal energy. Once you have trained for a while it is easy to govern your internal energies using your intention but it is impossible to do this when excited. If the Yi (意) is disturbed then it cannot govern the Qi and so your energy becomes scattered. An internal martial artist who becomes overly stimulated during combat is no longer an internal artist, as they will have to rely on brute physical power; a calm and focused mind is needed for internal energy control.

The negative aspect (perhaps it's negative anyway?) of this is that many people are addicted to adrenalin and the feeling of excitement that stress can produce for them. Some people may seek out extreme sports and activities in order to experience this excitement and we call these people 'adrenalin junkies'. Many people will gamble or take risks in their lives in order to generate the same 'buzz'. The majority of people will subconsciously seek out this same excitement through creating and getting involved in personal dramas within their romantic and interpersonal relationships. If these people engage with the processes inherent within the internal arts they will have this source of stimulation taken away from them. This is much better for their health, as their source of stimulation is actually draining their Kidneys, but they have to find contentment within states of perpetual centredness rather than extremes of excitement. These states are recommended by all ancient spiritual traditions but are not what many people are looking for in modern times.

For myself I can say that increasing my 'excitement threshold' has been a positive thing. Looking back at my younger years, it is clear for me to see that I, like many others, was addicted to the feelings of excitement that were produced in stressful situations. As is typical for teenagers and people in their 20s I created tensions and dramas within my life in order to generate the adrenalin-type experiences that I have now moved away from. In the beginning these dramas were created through relationships and then gradually through getting involved in confrontational and violent situations. As these states became more normal to me, the buzz was gone, and so recreational drugs replaced them.

As I moved further into my practice I changed the way in which my mind and body worked, thus moving me away from the extreme states of excitement (and of course their opposite, the extreme lows that came with them) that caused me to operate on an emotionally driven level. As I moved more into the centred state that allowed outside stresses to wash over me I came to generate more peace within my life. Once stress and drama have no addictive effect upon the body then they are no longer desirable and so trivial dramas become somewhat irrelevant. They are simply not needed and so you do not create them.

As in the case of the shooting in Thailand, there will always be random events within your life that are potentially risky. If you wish to experience life you have to accept that there will be dangers and sometimes situations will not be pleasant, but how you handle these situations will ultimately dictate how they affect you. If you can attain the state of centring the mind as discussed here then you are more likely to be able to deal with these situations in a calm and controlled manner... Just don't expect to ever be the life and soul of the next bungee jumping party you get invited to...

12

THE FA JIN CONTROVERSY
Damo Mitchell

Within the world of the internal martial arts, and more specifically Taijiquan, nothing brings with it as much controversy as the skill of Fa Jin (發勁). For those who do not know, Fa Jin can be translated as meaning to 'issue Jin'. The exact meaning of Jin is up for debate, but within my school we translate Jin as meaning 'the external expression of a force which originates within the body'.

Fa Jin and its exact application divides the Taijiquan world into two main groups – those who see Fa Jin as being nothing more than a description of the mechanical forces involved in grappling, and the second group who see Fa Jin as a way of uprooting an opponent with minimal to no muscular force. Those in the second group generally demonstrate the skill by lifting their partners into the air as if they were rag dolls – a feat that looks very impressive on video and in photos. Figure 12.1 shows this kind of Fa Jin usage, which can often look somewhat supernatural.

The argument against this kind of skill is that it appears almost superhuman, and those who have never felt it being applied to them do not believe that it is possible. Statements such as 'this only works on the weak-minded' and 'that would not work against a resistant opponent' are thrown around, and so the insults fly and the Taijiquan world is divided.

As a practitioner of Taijiquan who has experienced and trained in Fa Jin I feel that I have the right to have my own say on what exactly Fa Jin is. I am primarily from the second group – Fa Jin is a way of training to uproot an opponent through the use of minimal force to me. It is an important aspect of Taijiquan training, which unfortunately suffers much from the arguments and, as far as I see it, is both misunderstood and misrepresented by both groups, those for and those against its practice. Do not get me wrong though, I also enjoy grappling in Taijiquan and believe the training of both to be the most efficient way to develop martial skill.

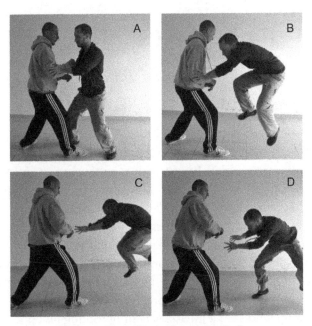

FIGURE 12.1: YANG TAIJIQUAN FA JIN

Figure 12.2 shows me using Fa Jin to uproot my training partner during a class in 2014.

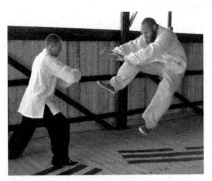

FIGURE 12.2: UPROOTING WITH FA JIN

The problem with Fa Jin is that it is generally seen and presented within a very limited viewpoint – it is either an undefeatable weapon or it is not. If you are stuck within this very limited viewpoint then there are always going to be problems with how this important aspect of Taijiquan practice is perceived. Do not misunderstand me though – it is not just those who are against this form of Fa Jin who cause this misperception, it is also those who practise and demonstrate it publicly. It is incorrect to perceive it purely as a martial weapon but also incorrect to sell it as the ultimate weapon. To keep it simple, it is a power development tool, a way of exploring structure and a method of learning how to read, absorb and then disrupt forces as they pass back and forth between two practitioners of the internal martial arts.

Fa Jin works by learning how to shape and stretch the soft tissues of the body in such a manner that they distribute mechanical pressures and forces from a point of contact down into the floor. As they do this they cause the Fa Jin issuer's body to move into a state of internal stress. This stress then reaches a certain peak before it releases this pressure back into the person applying force into the structure. As this happens there are a series of internal springs that are 'released' within the soft tissue structure of both the issuer and the receiver. The receiver of the force is then lifted up into the air by the force as their entire bodily structure is 'bounced' upwards away from the ground. The force of the spring within both parties' tissues then dictates just how high and far the 'bounce' is as the Fa Jin is issued outwards from the Taijiquan practitioner's body. This is all greatly enhanced by the practice of controlled relaxation and release. As the practitioner releases ever-increasing stored tensions within their body they drop more potential force into the elastic system they have created. There are far more complex aspects involved in the development of Jin within an art such as Taijiquan but this is a brief overview.

In order for this phenomenon to take place there have to be several factors in play. The first is that the issuer of the Jin (勁) needs to have trained their body to develop a clear line through to the floor whereby the force being applied into their body can be transferred down into the ground. Later this line is actually 'dissolved' and it is no longer needed, but it is vital in the early stages of practice. They then need to have built the various springs within the tissues through a lengthy process of stretching and relaxing the soft tissues of the body; generally, this is accomplished through prolonged practice of static postures. There then needs to be a clear line of force passed into their body from their partner/opponent. This force needs to be clear and direct, as if the person is giving them a prolonged push; it is this force that is then taken into the floor. The final aspect required to issue the Jin is that the target of the Jin has to have enough of an elastic structure within their own body for the release of the internal 'springs' to generate the uprooting force. If there is no structure within the target's body then the force is instead transferred into their skeletal structure. Instead of the target's soft tissues 'bouncing' them upwards into the air, they generally collapse instead as any weakness in their structure is exploited. It becomes an exit point for the power of the Jin being released into their body. Far from being visually impressive, this result is actually more realistically applied directly into competitive work. The 'bouncing' Fa Jin is something of a phenomenon generated between two practitioners of the internal arts or a similar body art that emphasises whole body connection and the use of soft tissues to shape the body into a single unit.

Figure 12.3 shows the various lines of force distribution and release involved in static Taijiquan training as well as in Fa Jin issuing.

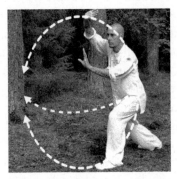

FIGURE 12.3: LINES OF FORCE DISTRIBUTION AND RELEASE

WHAT ARE THE USES OF FA JIN TRAINING?

Looking at the above description we can see that the impressive uprooting Fa Jin that causes so much controversy has a fairly limited scope of people with whom it can be used to dramatic visual effect. For this reason, it is important that internal martial arts practitioners do not see Fa Jin as a complete martial tool in its own right; for martial arts to be combat effective there must also be the practice of skills such as striking, footwork, grappling and so on. This is an important part of our own school for those interested in self-defence. Fa Jin is a separate skillset, which is vital to an art like Taijiquan's skill development, but its application is slightly more abstract outside of pushing hands drills. Below are some of the reasons why Fa Jin training is important within internal martial arts practice.

- As stated above, Fa Jin helps to train the elasticated strength of the soft tissues of the body and in particular the fascia. In Taijiquan they say that we should minimise 'Li' or brute muscular force. We should then train 'Jin', which is the force that can be developed deeper within the body's structure. Each time we issue or even receive Fa Jin into our body we are actually stressing and thus strengthening the lines of the body through which Jin travels. In this way we are helping to develop an internal strength that is more elasticated and spring-like than pure muscular power.

- The practice of Fa Jin helps to develop a very high level of physical sensitivity to incoming pressures. At first there needs to be a large degree of power put into your system to initiate the release of Jin, but with time the required pressures become less and less. At this time even the slightest push into your body will develop a series of internal changes within the tissues of the body that serve to redirect your force back into the opponent. Without Fa Jin practice your sensitivity to rapidly shifting pressures never really develops beyond a very low level.

- The practice of Fa Jin provides the platform from which the various internal forces of Taijiquan can be trained; these are namely Peng (掤), Lu (履), Ji (擠) and An (按) and their various derivatives. Translated as Wardoff, Rollback, Press and Push, these four powers are not simply ways to move your arms but rather different ways in which Jin can be directed through your connected body system in order to disrupt an opponent's structure. Without first learning to issue Fa Jin you cannot ever learn to place upon this Jin the 'characteristic' of one of these four qualities.

- Possibly the most important reason for learning how to issue Jin is that it is great fun. It is a way for two practitioners of pushing hands to apply and release pressures into each other's physical structure without the risk of injury. The level of skill of these practitioners then dictates which person is uprooted away from the other. In gaining skill through this friendly exchange you will find that many of the internal skills of Taijiquan, such as effective rooting, are improved. If you ever have the chance to push hands with somebody much better than yourself, you will have the chance to experience how just about any weakness in your structure results in you being uprooted from the floor and 'bounced' away.

The skills developed through this practice are then applied into more unstructured and competitive martial work for those who wish to see how Fa Jin is put into combative training. At this stage the impressive 'bouncing' feats you see in videos such as those pictured earlier are not so common, as a competitive opponent will rarely be foolish enough to give you the clean, straight push that is required to touch upon the 'springs' within their body. Since the floor is more difficult to touch, you will instead find that the skills of the Jins you have developed will manifest in more subtle ways as you are able to touch their root more cleanly, manipulate their structure and absorb their force without resisting it in any way. All of these are skills that any true martial arts practitioner will instantly recognise the value of.

In conclusion, I believe that Fa Jin of this kind has been misunderstood by those who do not practise it and misrepresented by many who do. It is a drill like any other and a single skillset that should form a part of any classical Taijiquan practice regime. Look to any videos of masters in China or refer to stories of those who lived prior to the invention of the camera and you will find that they all practise and demonstrate this kind of force. The problem is simply that through the lens of the rather two-dimensional modern/Western mind Fa Jin is difficult to understand. It is a more circular mental approach that is required in order to understand the value and meaning of Fa Jin training.

Ultimately though, it should be remembered that it is up to each and every one of us what we practise. We never really have the right to become angry at what others do or pass negative comments upon an entire aspect of the internal arts simply because we do not like it. Each person's practice is their own, and as long as they are not 'selling' a skillset as something more than it is then they are doing nobody any harm. We should all focus on our own practice, and if you don't like something…simply don't do it.

13

QI GONG, TANTRA AND GHOSTS

Damo Mitchell

Confusion has arisen in modern times, as we have now been widely exposed to the teachings of both Yoga and the Daoist arts. Both of these systems present different views of how we as humans function beyond the level of physical form. This is due to the systems' individual aims and focuses. The Daoist internal arts initially focus heavily upon the energetic realm, whilst Yoga seems to discuss the spiritual/consciousness realm to a far higher degree. There is a very good reason for this. This reason is Tantra (तन्त्र).

In modern times the term Tantra is often equated with sexual practices. The alternative community has turned what was originally the study of the energy body into a way to heighten sexual pleasure under the illusion that this will lead to spiritual elevation. Tantra was not originally majorly concerned with sexual practices, as only a very small part of its teachings concerned dual-cultivation methods of this sort. The term Tantra can be translated as meaning 'gaining understanding through expansion of the awareness'; it was originally the study of expanding the frequencies of our comprehension in order to study the more subtle energy realms that sat beyond the physical body. Being a Sanskrit term it was originally a branch of the Yogic school's practice and could basically be equated with Qi Gong. Any form of energy work including Qi Gong, Dao Yin (導引) or even internal alchemy would fall under the bracket of Tantric practices. Tantra was Yoga's way of studying the energy body.

It is rare to find a Tantric Yoga school these days. Many may well say that they are practising Tantra when they are not. If you have the chance to witness an authentic Yogic Tantric school practising you will see that many of their exercises essentially look like Qi Gong. After the performance of Asanas (आसन), which are the physical exercises most modern people would equate with Yoga, Tantric Yoga practitioners often sit and breathe whilst making particular hand postures, chanting and moving their fingers and arms around in time with their breath to shift Qi, which we can equate with Prana (प्राण) along the length of the meridians, which we can equate with Nadi (नाडी). Tantric Yogis often work with three key energy centres in their body, which correspond to the location of the Dan Tien, and refine frequencies inside of their bodies to lift Jing into Qi and then into Shen; in short they are practising their own form of Qi Gong. Many of these Tantric practices were passed on to the Buddhists of Tibet, and now there are also Tantric schools of Buddhist Yoga coming from this tradition as well.

At some point Tantra was largely removed from Yoga, leaving many schools with a bridge that could not be crossed. Students were now trying to jump from Asanas (physical body work) to meditation on the Chakra (चक्र) (spiritual body work), which cannot easily be done. You cannot simply move from physical body work to the spirit body – it is too big a jump. There must be some kind of energetic practice that bridges the two.

Part of the reason why Tantra was removed from Yogic schools was because of its connection to the realm of ghosts and hungry spirits. Work with Qi is, to some extent, also connecting us to other realms not normally available to those who are operating on a purely physical level. When we access the energy body and work with it for a long time it becomes clear that not only is the realm of Qi a bridge to the realm of divine spirit, but it also connects us to the world of spiritual entities that can either be benevolent, neutral or malignant. This is the reason for many cases of spiritual possession and madness that are the result of energy work. Travelling extensively within the Far East has opened my eyes to the way in which these cultures embrace the concept of spiritual entities with great ease. Every day in places such as Thailand, India or Bali local people go to the nearest temple to appease the spirits before going to their offices to work. Exorcisms are carried out regularly, and there is no doubt within people's minds that spirits live alongside us throughout the course of our daily lives. Within Tantric schools it was believed that the risks of opening the energy body and mind up to the invasion of spiritual entities was too great and so it was gradually phased out of the practices except for in the case of high-level adepts. Now the bridge was broken and no work could be carried out on the level of consciousness without great difficulty and, arguably, natural talent. What was left was often physical practice based around improving the health of the body. From here numerous other styles were born, each focusing upon bodily purification in a different manner, whilst the original aim of working towards conscious elevation was generally forgotten or relegated to the level of intellectual study.

There may be some subjects in the above paragraph that some find hard to fathom. Belief in spirits, either positive or negative, is not something that sits comfortably with the belief systems of many in the West. Whether or not this is the case, it is kind of irrelevant, as this was the belief system of those who founded the systems of Yoga and Qi Gong, so therefore anything created within these systems will take this belief into consideration. The spirit world would always have been a factor for the ancient sages. Another facet inherent within the Yogic systems, rarely discussed now, is the development of Siddhis (सिद्धि) or abilities similar to the abilities developed from prolonged practice of the Daoist arts. These are abilities such as increased levels of intuition, telepathy, the ability to control others' thoughts and movements and so on. These abilities were associated with the opening of the Dan Tien or the seven spinal fires within Daoism (influenced by Tantric Buddhist systems) and with awakening of the seven Chakra within Hinduism. Many of these skills were then discussed elementally as well as within the Tantric traditions. For the teachers of Tantra each element came with a different skill, such as the following.

- Water: The ability to transmit healing information into water so that it could be drunk as medicine. Also, the ability to control water in others' bodies, thus making them move around according to your will — essentially a skillset similar to what is known as Kong Jin (空勁) or 'empty force' within Daoism. Tantric Yoga teachers would teach the physical movements of their systems in this manner.

- Fire: Tantric masters of fire could generate warmth from their hands and even set objects alight simply by using their intention.

- Earth: These practitioners could, to some degree, control their own physicality. A test for them would be to place their hand lightly onto solid rock and leave a deep handprint. This is a phenomenon well recorded, even in relatively recent times, in Tibet.

- Air: This is the element of the mind, and those Tantric masters at this level could control the thoughts, beliefs and emotions of other people.

- Void: The final element is the divine element of emptiness, and those at this level could bring on experiences of stillness for other people at will. This could lead to high-level healings and mental awakenings.

The above elementally related skills are linked to each Chakra, excluding the first two, meaning that those with an awakened Chakra are classically said to be able to manifest the above abilities. Those who could not do this had not reached the stage of working effectively with their Chakra and were required to practise more. Is it these skills that are the reason for the removal of Tantra from the Yogic school? Did the ancient teachers really want the majority of people to have access to these abilities? I have met some teachers who can manifest this sort of ability, and in my experience they do not have to be particularly nice people. The connection between virtuous manifestation of compassion and development of high-level skills does not really exist as you would expect. Sadly, you can be a jerk and still develop real internal power over people.

Daoism and the internal arts that came out of the tradition, such as Qi Gong, had the opposite problem. The body work and energy work were kept. This presented a solid bridge to move into the energetic realm, but almost every school dropped the spirit body practices. This was largely due to the fact that most internal schools went down the medical path, and working with the consciousness on this level was not required for repairing and maintaining a person's health. This means that many practitioners of Qi Gong are stuck at the level of the energy body and cannot progress, as very few esoteric Daoist schools still maintain their teachings on the spirit body. Those schools that do this class themselves as religious, wisdom or spiritual schools of Daoism rather than medical schools, which we tend to have more contact with in the West.

This brings us to internal alchemy, which is the form of sitting meditation most commonly practised by Daoists in modern times.

Alchemy can basically be divided into two main schools of thought. The first school is aiming to develop a spiritual form of the self in order to attain immortality; this is known as developing the spiritual embryo. The second school does not aim for this and instead aims for complete emptiness and merging with the Dao, thus converting ever-higher frequencies of energetic substances into a state whereby it connects with the frequency of Heaven.

In the form of alchemy aiming to convert Jing into Qi and then into Shen there comes a point when complete emptiness is attained. This is the same experience discussed within many Buddhist and Hindu schools whereby one dissolves the physical form and the mind to just leave complete connection with the universe. For many this is a ground-breaking experience and a life-defining moment, myself included. It corresponds to the stage of linking your own spiritual energy, via the Chong Mai (衝脈), into the vastness of Wuji (无极) so that you experience the stillness at your own core. The majority of my own practice these days is around this kind of work, and my own exploration for authentic teachers is around the subject of alchemy. The problem with this kind of work, and many who have experienced the same will most likely agree, is staying here. These glimpses of connection to a profound state tend to be fleeting. Whilst the experiences bring some kind of change to a person's outlook on existence, it is difficult to remain here for long periods of time. The reason for this is because these are simply glimpses of direct contact with the consciousness body; we are touching upon the next stage in our inner development but are not yet able to fully progress to this stage. This is partly because the foundational work within the energy body is not yet completed; the energetic stage is a long process that cannot be skipped, as we will be left with the problem of never really understanding or refining our own consciousness.

Why discuss this? Because I think it is important to look at these issues if we ever wish to use any of the internal arts to progress beyond the most fundamental of levels. First, in the West we need to develop more respect for the inherent risks involved in powerful energy work. If we are going to engage in practices such as this, then guidelines should be adhered to and advice should be sought in order to prevent any illnesses occurring, whether energetically or spiritually. It is a constant problem that the arrogance of modern practitioners is that they seem to think they can take ancient Eastern practices and simply adapt them to suit their purposes, throwing out the bits that they 'don't believe in' simply because they incorrectly view ancient cultures as primitive. Second, we must also understand that many of the systems we are presented with today have been changed in this way. Pieces are missing, and a great deal of searching is most likely required by those who really want to delve deep into internal cultivation. Please note that I am not trying to be negative about either Yoga or Qi Gong; I think both are amazing systems with the potential to lead people towards high levels of comprehension. I am just discussing the way they are currently being practised. For me, I have always trusted in classical teachings, whether verbal or written within classical texts. I work on the reasoning that the people who put the classical teachings together were most likely far more wise than I, so I should probably listen to them, even if their reasoning and belief systems are currently lost to me. In short, I operate through trust.

14

TAIJIQUAN AND EVOLUTION

Paul Mitchell

Taijiquan, be it the grand ultimate fist or the boxing style that uses the motive force of creation, is my life's study. Okay, as a martial artist, all martial arts and much more are my study, but for me there are no limits to the principles contained within the forms of Taijiquan. Training to be a person with no limits is for me what the study of martial arts is all about.

I think that before I become immersed in this written piece, I should attempt to define my definition of the study of the martial arts. To the uninitiated and also possibly some who consider that a purely academic approach to all things internal is even remotely possible, the study of martial arts may seem a competitive, brutal, basic person's way. This is simply not the case.

The study of the martial way (as opposed to that of martial sports) is the study of contentious issues. For this reason, many avoid its rigours, and for the main part it is populated by the physically tough but, unfortunately, emotionally immature. My personal opinion is that, again unfortunately, in modern times egos rule the day and any notion of philosophy loses out to raging hormones, mainly testosterone. In these times Western sports science has filtered into the martial arts; a supposed martial artist is measured by the amount of trophies that he/she has accumulated in their youth. This is, unfortunately, the nature of sport and arguably the blueprint for modern societies' design. I cannot see this situation improving any day soon, but I have long not cared what others do and I always endeavour to both commit my study to what I consider to be the deeper elements of martial arts and subsequently teach it accordingly.

If studied correctly, the external methods, being those that involve muscular engagement for the proliferation of punches, kicks, blocks, chokes, throws and the like, teach the individual many things that are all but impossible to learn in any other way. Thirty-five years in I still remember the clumsy awkward man in his mid-20s who walked into the dojo for the first time. He, or I, was not a particularly sophisticated individual, but if I compare myself and my understanding of life with most people at the time and am honest in a non-arrogant or self-effacing manner, I was certainly not stupid by comparison. I was certainly clumsy, awkward and unable to move in a coordinated manner. These are the first lessons to be learned by any aspiring martial artist.

Of course these rather basic skills can be learned in an arguably more complex and aesthetically pleasing manner by learning to dance, but nobody is attacking the wannabe dancer. Learning to keep your head whilst under the pressure of someone attacking you certainly assists in the whole live-in-the-moment-focus thing.

Dropping the mind and breath into the belly, again whilst under pressure, changes a person. In time these moments of pressure, as pressure does, cause personal growth. Dealing with bare, blistered feet on a hard floor, and sometimes being thrown onto the same, causes the normal discomforts of life to dull by comparison, whilst a degree of suffering most definitely brings out a feeling of compassion for those of any species that are truly suffering.

In time this uncomfortable lifestyle choice ceases to be one of discomfort and the time in the dojo feels like peace incarnate.

To summarise, I would say that the skills learned whilst studying the external martial arts revolve around physical strength and coordination, self-defence, self-realisation, relationships with others and eventually compassion for yourself and all living entities. How long does this take? For me a long time, but I am a slow learner, so it is most likely an individual thing. Let's face it, in such things we don't all start in the same place.

There comes a time in all people's lives when the things of youth must or should be surrendered gracefully. Please don't get me wrong and imagine that I am about to write that a person should surrender to the onslaught of time and the ageing process and give up the martial way. Most do I am afraid. This to me is one of the differences between a martial art and a martial sport. As in all sports the player is over the hill by the time they are in their early 30s. In martial arts we do not play. Games are for the amusement of children; instead the study of our art continues until the moment of our demise. Now, as I am not yet at that moment, gladly I have to say, I cannot predict that I shall sustain the daily or even minute-to-minute enthusiasm to continue my path of choice until the precise moment of my death, but I intend to give it my best shot. Sports people peak and trough; artists mature with time.

So what is it that a martial artist should do (as I and a damn good poem alluded to) in order to surrender gracefully with the cessation of their youthful vigour? For the answer to this question we must look to the example set for us by the sporting fraternity. We must ask ourselves why we don't see older sprinters, jumpers, javelin throwers or even boxers. The exception seems to be marathon runners. I am definitely no expert on the marathon, as it pertains to running, but it seems likely to me that the mind plays a major role in the marathon run – good breath, good posture and clear mind are almost the required requisites for the marathon study of the martial arts.

In the youthful world of the competitive sports person, the will to win must dominate the very soul of the competitor if they are to finish ahead of the crowd. In the young, maybe this attitude is all well and good – some would say necessary, but not I. It is this competitive nature that makes it possible for our young to be dragged by the evil of our leaders into wars that just lead to suffering and despair.

As a martial artist ages and matures this naïve, non-questioning and almost headlong behaviour is obviously not desirable. This is the point where meditation should start to take a major role in a person's study. In this way the follower of the martial way has evolved by almost shedding the skin of their former testosterone-driven self and begun the journey into the next evolutionary version of themselves. In a footnote to this, my last statement, I would have to say that having over the years assisted several females of our species through the rocky waters of the external arts, they are far wiser by nature than their male counterparts.

Physically, as our bodies age we burn off our life energy. We only have to look at the people who live a long life to realise that all but the very few have not overdone anything, be it eating, drinking, sexual activity or even hard physical exercising. In short, we wear ourselves out by our behaviour.

It is for this reason that I write that at some stage the studies of a martial artist must again evolve this time from a predominantly external and physical system into a predominantly internal and mind-orientated one. As I attempt to pick my techniques carefully in combat, so I also attempt to pick my words when I both talk and write. I used the word predominantly when I stated that I felt a martial artist should evolve from external to internal as they aged. In truth, we should never leave a stage of our development behind, and to sacrifice the physical for the energetic completely seems to me to be akin to sacrificing a quality of life for a quantity of the same. Okay, it may be best if at about 60 we did just a little light physical exercise whilst meditating and periodically climbing to our feet for some light Qi Gong exercises. Personally, I would sooner die a few years earlier but keep a good degree of my accumulated physical strength and persona. As all things in life, this issue is about balance for me.

Having made the conscious decision to evolve into the energetic aspects of the martial arts, the first problem is to find a teacher who has the required knowledge and the ability to pass said knowledge on to you. It is often stated that one of the hardest things to find in the martial world is a good teacher; it is then also often said that it is even harder to find a good student. It is little more than a miracle that certainly the internal martial arts have survived at all. But as is the way of men, survived they have, albeit in small pockets.

It is, unfortunately, my experience that many if not most teachers of Taijiquan fall into the categories of either believing that all is physical and those who say otherwise are all using smoke and mirrors or simply teaching slow, rhythmic movements in time with breathing for health reasons.

The first category often appeals to what I rather disparagingly refer to as the meathead fraternity in the martial arts community. They simply play to the crowd and often do very nicely for themselves due to the fact that they have a large potential clientele. Unfortunately, these teachers can be quite defensive due to the fact that there are plenty of examples of internal force being demonstrated on social media and this has the potential to threaten their livelihood due to their lack of ability in such matters.

I personally do not mind the second category because they fill a need. Okay, what they teach lacks a certain depth, and I have come to realise that authentic Taijiquan is not for everyone, but if people can at least reap some of its benefits through this simplified method, all is good.

To the completely uninitiated amongst us in terms of the concept of the internal arts, all this can be a little confusing, but we were all at this stage at some point, albeit in this life or a previous one.

If I was to say that technically in an external system a martial artist uses muscle, bone, gravity and leverage against an attacker or opponent whereas an internal exponent uses fascia lines, soft tissues, vital or internal energy and mental intent, I would not be doing the subject justice, but I would be pointing you in the right direction.

I know all this sounds most combative and almost – a word I really like – pugilistic, but in truth, by the time a martial artist has reached the stage in his/her evolutionary journey that this transition is the natural and correct course of action, the conflicts within them are all but resolved. They have made friends with their own worst enemy: themselves. In short, they have found that place of peace within themselves.

On a personal level, all martial arts are about self-defence. I say on a personal level because ultimately they are really about the bigger picture, and within that it is fairly obvious that personal well-being or indeed survival are not of paramount importance. Self-defence is a large concept. It is often assumed by non-martial artists that people of my persuasion are a paranoid bunch with the idea that there is a potential attacker around every corner. Whilst this is not true in the sense of there necessarily being a masked attacker waiting to pounce with a weapon in hand, who can deny that our futures are uncertain and a heightened state of awareness is a wise precaution against calamities, whatever form they may take?

Our most likely attackers that will eventually kill the vast majority of us are sickness and disease or eventually just the running out of time. There is no escaping these most persistent adversaries, but we can most certainly draw the battle lines and take them on in our own territory. In this way the health aspects of the study of Taijiquan are just a further development of the martial aspect and as such still come under the umbrella term of martial arts.

So now to the uninitiated reader it may well seem that I am fighting shy of the obviously awkward task of laying before them how an internal martial art works if not by muscular contraction, leverage or even gravity. Shy I am not.

The first hurdle that a newbie to the internal studies must overcome, having been fortunate enough to find a teacher with the right qualities in order to guide them through the somewhat confusing process of the inward journey, is that of their own mind. Certainly, for people who have spent long and arduous years in the study of the external martial arts, there is a tendency to be suspicious of anything that cannot be seen, touched or otherwise proved to be factual by one of our physical senses.

Obviously, a degree of scepticism in all matters esoteric is a healthy and necessary thing. A good teacher in the internal arts should have the ability to demonstrate in various ways that they have some abilities that could be attributed to a personal control over their internal aspects, but in truth most at the beginning could be attributed to smoke and mirrors. It is for this reason that the new student needs to open their mind and give their practice their all for a reasonable period of time. Having spent a few months of training with periods of daily personal practice, the new trainee will discover energetic realms within themselves that will cause any doubts that they may have encountered in their initial studies to dissolve. At this stage the mind of the student begins to open and the possibilities for them to achieve their true potential come to the fore.

It is understandably common for people who begin a study of Taijiquan to assume that the movements or form that has become a fairly common commodity for advertisers to use in order to sell their wares from music videos to painkillers is Taijiquan. This is not the case. In Daoist theory Taijiquan is the spiralling energy that is the basis for all existence. The word 'Quan' (拳) means fist or can be taken to mean martial art. Taijiquan as such is often referred to as the motive force of creation. For these reasons the term Taijiquan is maybe best translated as the martial art or the boxing style that uses the motive force of creation.

From this the reader can no doubt deduce that the Taiji form is merely the vehicle by which the practitioner is first manipulated by this motive force and in time learns to turn the tables and manipulate it instead.

It is necessary for an individual who wishes to embrace all aspects of Taijiquan to begin the study of Nei Gong. I would assume that most readers of this piece are aware of what this entails. Therefore, it is probably not necessary for me to explain my previous assertion beyond saying that a high degree of internal awareness and eventually control are an imperative requisite for a deep study of Taijiquan.

In many physical activities from sports to dancing there is a new buzz term – fascia lines. These have come to be understood to have the potential by sports technologists to increase the strength and connected movement of an athlete without the massive burn off of energy created by the use of oxygen in the contraction of the human muscular system. I think it is true to say that this information was first gleaned within the Taiji community.

Taijiquan makes particular use of these fascia lines. They are often referred to as the Jing Jin (經筋) lines or connective tissues. The Western medical profession is also just beginning to realise the significance of the, as they term it, 'bio fascia system'. Previously, doctors simply thought that it was a bag-like organ that laid beneath the skin. I don't really know what, if any, function they believed it to fulfil – possibly a protective layer.

This bio fascia or connective tissue system as I understand it is in terms of placement in the human body rather like the pith of an orange, and not only lies beneath the peel, or in the case of the human body the skin, but also runs through to the very core.

In the practice of Taijiquan the connective tissues play many major roles. First, although when the human muscles are engaged they contract, this has a limited if any usage for the movements or postures of Taijiquan. Unlike the gross muscular system, the fascia system expands when engaged. This expansion gives the human form a tensile strength far beyond the potential of the muscular system. It is a misnomer that whilst a person is performing the Taijiquan form they are relaxed in a, for want of a better word, floppy or disconnected way. The Taijiquan form is often referred to as steel wrapped in cotton or sometimes silk. The gross or large muscle groups hang from the skeletal structure as the connective tissues are engaged and therefore expanded, giving the practitioner the potential power of tensile steel.

The second role of these connective tissue lines revolves around the fact that they are known to carry energy rather like fibre optics and are often referred to as the riverbed of the meridians. It was inevitable that at some point in my present ramble I was going to get to the stage whereby I had to bring our meridian system into the mix. This next section may sound a little out there if you have little or no real knowledge of the internal arts. In the practice of Taijiquan, or I should say the Taijiquan that I practise, because as in all things I cannot speak or indeed write for anyone else, we use a particular hand position often referred to as the 'fair maiden's hand'. This hand position is concave in nature with the joints open, giving it a, once again, connected feeling that runs throughout our whole body. As its name suggests, this hand position has a distinctly gentle feel to it. It may surprise you when I state that this is our martial hand.

Before I continue with my assertions about the role of the meridians and also our almost feminine grip whilst performing our Taijiquan form and indeed any partner work that we may engage in, it is necessary for me to expand a little (no pun intended) on the nature of our connective tissues.

These connective tissues also include our ligaments and our soft tissues. Those of you who have engaged in the practices of standing in both 'Wuji' and 'Zhan Zhuang' (站樁) will I am sure be acquainted with the idea of dissolving the soft tissues down to the arches of the feet. Some, if not most, of you will no doubt be aware that at some stage of the proceedings we are waiting to experience through 'ting' (listening) an equal and opposite return wave of what is generally referred to as Peng.

This 'Peng wave' that rises from the earth up through our 'bubbling spring' point on the soles of our feet is the mechanism that we use both to engage and transmit throughout our connective tissues.

At this point I shall return to our 'fair maiden's hands'. The Taijiquan classics state that amongst other things:

> The internal energy is rooted beneath our feet, comes forth through our legs, is controlled by our centre and functions through our fingers. From feet to legs, legs to the waist, all should operate as one unit. By acting as a unit, it is possible to expand or contract with precise timing to suit the situation.

So, from our feet to our centre. Obviously, our energetic centre lies in our lower Dan Tien. In other words, the energetic pulse that has travelled from the earth up through the meridians in our legs gathers in the lower Dan Tien. From there it travels with a little help from our 'Yi' or deep intention mind to, as the classics say, our fingers.

At this point in the proceedings a practitioner feels as if his/her fingertips are electrodes. The soft, light grip of the hands as they make contact with another's body touches into the depth of their fascia or connective tissues. At this moment, due to the fact that the connective tissues are as I stated previously the riverbed of the meridians, there is a merging of both meridian systems and we have almost hacked into the energy system of the other party.

A common question from beginners, when demonstrating this by affecting the receiver's form or root, is understandably along the lines of: can you affect anybody in this way?

I think that in order to answer this question we must consider what the demonstration of the external expression of internal force is about in terms of the development of the Taijiquan exponent. First, it is not, in my opinion, a replacement for physical methods of self-defence. In other words, if a person who has learned to defend themselves physically is attacked by a marauding, axe-wielding maniac they should, just as the moment is most definitely fixing them in the physical realm, deal with the situation physically. The run-like-hell principle should be applied if at all possible. If escape is not feasible, second, pick up a bigger weapon like a chair. If both these options are unavailable for any reason, use simple direct action in order to survive. It is definitely true that one should not attempt to use any form of internal skill against life-threatening attack.

So having ascertained when not to use internal skills, let's try to put them into perspective. I mentioned earlier that a person who feels they may have the will and determination to go along with their wish to attain the deeper skillsets that are possible to attain through a dedicated study of Taijiquan should be also studying Nei Gong. A person who studies Nei Gong goes through a process, referred to as the Nei Gong process. Within this process they develop internal awareness of their Dan Tien and meridian system and eventually control of these elements of themselves. Again, I would imagine that most people who are reading this or have had their interest held to this point are aware of the complexities of the Nei Gong process. For the uninitiated, I will simply state that fairly near to the beginning of this process a new trainee has their lower Dan Tien awoken from its semi-dormant state that is the norm for a mature human being. When this occurs the recipient becomes energised, and it is at this point that their meridian system begins to be open enough for the free flow of their internal energy and subsequent inflow of another person's. Suddenly this does not sound so pugilistic I think.

There are elements of Taijiquan principles that are connected with the connective tissues that can be used for martial arts against, for want of a better word, an unsophisticated attacker, but these methods are almost too easy to apply to put them down in words for general consumption. One of the often-asked questions in martial art circles revolves around whether there are indeed 'secrets' or secret techniques or principles. Many teachers of both external and internal martial arts would likely answer in the negative. Personally, I would not agree with them.

Some of what I have attempted to explain in this chapter would by some be viewed as things that should be kept secret. Again, it is my personal opinion that although what I have written is easy enough to understand by a person with a degree of the groundwork having been achieved, the theory is one thing and the practice most certainly another. In other words, there are no short cuts, and understanding must be the beginning of intense practice if anything of value is to be achieved.

The skills that must be kept secret are the simple ones that are relatively easy to gain proficiency in. If a student achieves skills that are perceived by them, and more relevantly in their early development other people, as important, their ego can become inflated and further development is all but impossible for them to achieve. There is an old Chinese saying that I quite like that states: 'When the ego goes, the chi comes.' On a physical level this simple statement implies that it is not until a person can go 'Sung' or relax their tissues completely whilst using the achieved 'Peng' wave to expand their structure, having previously been successful in their endeavours to reach a fairly high level of Nei Gong practice, that the ability to transmit to another person is possible.

In this process it is not possible to dissolve all residual tension from out of the human body whilst still being controlled by low-level consciousness (the ego), such as greed, envy or resentment, or even harbouring a competitive nature. Therefore, when the ego goes, the chi comes.

There is most certainly a benefit to be gained by practitioners of Nei Gong from the inclusion of partner work in their practices. Whilst standing in 'Wuji' or 'Zhan Zhuang' a practitioner will routinely dissolve their soft tissues down to the arches of their feet. In this manner the individual is said to be 'rooting'.

Rooting is a basic skill of a practitioner of Taijiquan. Whilst rooting, a person should be able to take physical pressure (a push) against their body. It is my experience that the majority of people who 'root' cannot achieve this without having been tested in this manner. In effect, they are not actually achieving 'root' and their practice is therefore fruitless in this particular element. However, it is also my experience that this skill is in most cases relatively easily achieved through the manner I have just outlined.

It is often stated that Taijiquan as a martial system specialises in yielding. I do not personally like this statement, as it can be misleading. Yielding as a word implies to me that a person moves backwards away from their partner as pressure is applied. This is not so, and if we were to substitute the word 'absorb' for that of 'yield' we would, I think, be getting closer to the truth.

Having had pressure from their training partner's push applied to their body, the skilled Taijiquan practitioner uses this pressure to add to the mass that they sink to their foot arches. As there is always an equal and opposite reaction, this added mass increases the returned Peng wave and consequently the emission of internal force is magnified proportionally. Simple, eh? As always, understanding is one thing and achievement another.

I think it is relatively obvious from what I have written in this chapter about the evolution that is achievable from moving from the external martial arts to the internal methods that the acquisition of internal force is not primarily about physical self-defence against a human being or indeed multiples of the same. Having said that, there are many advantages to be gained through the internal studies that readily cross back over to the external martial arts. Just as we are holistic beings, so too are our artistic abilities.

Unlike physical skills, internal ones increase with time and the ageing process. We can from this maybe glean a little about the mindset of those who formulated the internal arts such as Taijiquan so very long ago. All the skills learned by the study of the external martial arts are encapsulated in the internal methods but, I would say, in a far more cranial way. It is also true that whilst engaged in external combat there is obviously a very real presence of danger in the shape of possible physical damage to both parties. It seems likely to me that the internal methods of combat fitted well into the mindset of older, very skilled martial artists so that they could continue with their life's studies and endeavours without inflicting or having inflicted upon them physical damage as their bodies aged and lost some degree of their recuperative ability.

There are so many other elements and advantages to the sincere study of Taijiquan but this chapter is already twice as long as I intended. As always, good training my friends.

15

ON BEING A MISERABLE BASTARD

Damo Mitchell

A couple of years ago I was in Hong Kong training in the internal arts as well as receiving treatment for an injured shoulder. Whilst there I had some free time, so I wandered around the city and took the chance to see the protests taking place in the centre of the island around the Wan Chai district. Thousands of the Hong Kong people had taken to the streets in protest against the Chinese government's political stance with regards to Hong Kong's independence. It was good to wander around and meet some of the people involved in the 'occupy central' movement. The area of the protest I was involved in had something of a party atmosphere and I had a lot of fun being a part of the general dissent on the streets.

This is the kind of experience I enjoy: people finding ways to express their individuality and opinions whilst coming together for a purpose. The beauty of it is the passion that comes to the surface: a bubbling up of people's inner beliefs, which generates a heady energy that is great to be a part of. It is this kind of self-expression that gives off the energy I enjoy, and in many ways it is the same kind of energy manifested within a class of people training in the internal arts. This is the art, the essence and the meaning of training to me, and it is this that I have dedicated myself to training in and teaching others to find. In this way it is possible to end two of the most uninspiring aspects of human nature: apathy and an obsession with triviality.

The search for escape from the mundane is probably the closest I can say that I ever come to having 'fun'. I say the closest I ever come, as I don't really understand the term 'fun'. What does this mean, and why are most people so obsessed with tapping into this emotion?

I am sure that some reading this are already repeating within their head the same thing I have been told whenever I have asked this question out loud: 'What a miserable bastard!' This is completely wrong though. I am far from miserable; I just don't need fun in my life.

It is a mistake that many people seem to believe that there are two basic states in life – not having fun and having fun. I used to think this when I was younger, and so I divided my life like so. I would work and carry out all the mundane tasks in my life that needed doing and then as soon as I was free I headed out and looked for 'fun'. This usually revolved around going to a pub or party or mixing with friends. Over time I realised that this was actually quite dull, and so my 'not having fun' state started to cross over into my 'having fun' state. In order to relieve the boredom I sought to make the 'fun' more extreme and so drugs were added to the mix. This gave me a temporary respite from the constant state of boredom, as I had a sudden peak in the enjoyment of my free time.

Over time once again my mind started to 'normalise' this state of enjoyment and so my life started to level out again. I believe that this is what happens to many people in their lives, and so the body's need for more extreme versions of fun increases and increases. You are literally building up your tolerance for fun, meaning that the highs start to vanish from your state of being. This leaves you with two basic choices – lead a life of seeking out more extreme versions of fun (which usually revolve around self-destructive behaviour) or settling for a mundane life of triviality devoid of any major periods of enjoyment – something we often euphemise to some degree by naming it 'growing up'. Now that flat state of constancy has been reached, you are supposed to start seeking meaning in your life through climbing the corporate ladder, having a family or adding to your accumulated wealth and belongings. Don't get me wrong – if you have a burning desire to do these things then go ahead, that's fine. Just make sure that you are not doing them on societally programmed auto-drive.

On a personal level all of the above sound kind of pointless to me. It is a state of natural emotional evolution that I recognised somewhere deep down inside from a relatively young age, and so for this reason I decided to step away from 'fun seeking' long ago.

In lieu of making my life about temporary highs I instead sought to give my life some kind of purpose and tap into the energy of self-expression, which I found to give my life so much more value. In the same way that an artist may paint or sculpt to express the energy inside of their heart, I studied the internal arts as a way to bring this energy out into my direct environment. Through personal cultivation this energy can then be helped to evolve and then re-expressed outwards to make a constantly changing art form that is manifested through my mind, body and energetic system. Though I shy away from using the word 'fun', I would have to say that it comes pretty close. The only difference is that it does not 'normalise' in the same way that many external sources of pleasure do, and so there is no dropping back into the lows of 'non-enjoyment' that many people experience all too often. With constant training and evolution I have definitely begun to find that my training ultimately makes me more 'simple' in my wants and needs. The energy expressed also becomes simpler and simpler, something that I feel brings a deep-rooted feeling of contentment – a state far preferable to 'fun' for me.

I believe that going through your extremes of highs and lows eventually leads to that central point where self-expression becomes stagnated. Your internal energy can no longer be easily tapped into and thus you run the risk of becoming a person running on 'autopilot' for this whole life. This leads to a lack of passion and – in the case of your own beliefs – apathy. How many times do we hear people say things like 'I used to be so passionate when I was younger' or 'When I was young I really thought I could change the world'? Again, this change of heart is often put down to simply 'growing up' when in fact it is because you built too high a 'fun tolerance' through your seeking of constant highs to escape the lows. Your inner energy can no longer be felt, self-expression is gone and any kind of fuelled passion for anything is far out of your reach. Apathy is merely spiritual distance from the energy of your Heart.

This was what was beautiful about the protests in Hong Kong. On the television they showed mostly footage of tear gas and violent clashes, when in fact my experience of the protests was large groups of people tapping into the energy of their self-expression, shedding their apathy and getting away from the autopilot mode that drives society. I saw faces lit up with life and beauty as energy flowed through the crowds. If you have ever spent much time in Hong Kong, or any similar city like London or Washington DC, you will know how rare it is to see the general public looking beautifully lit up with energy and passion rather than simply going about the humdrum of their normal daily lives.

My confusion with people's ideas of fun has often caused me difficulty. These difficulties are generally around what are socially accepted sources of fun. These socially accepted forms of fun generally revolve around social dinners, after-dinner games or maybe going out to restaurants for a chit-chat and catching up with people. I often find that I am pressured into these kinds of events where it is expected that you sit down with people you have not seen in a while and make small talk about their lives or their children. As you do this you make polite comments about the food you are eating and occasionally resort to discussing the weather if any awkward silences arise. Once you have chatted, which usually means telling other people about the things you have done lately and listening to them do the same, you go on your way and quickly forget everything that was said. By the next day everything goes back to normal and essentially the social event becomes yet another waste of time that you will never get back. Time that could have been better spent training.

The difficulty I have with these kinds of events is the lack of fairness. If you try to avoid these kinds of events you are labelled miserable and rude and run the risk of offending many people. This is because you have tried to avoid a socially acceptable form of 'fun', something that should never be done. Why I say that this is unfair is because you can never impose your open sense of 'fun' onto these same people if it is not one of the socially accepted forms of 'fun', a form of enjoyment taken from the rather short list of 'fun things humans do'. For example, Qi Gong practice for many is not considered enjoyable. Meditation would never be something that many people consider as a pleasurable way to spend their evening. So if I were to suggest to those around me (excluding those who train in the internal arts) that they all come over one evening and we practise meditation together for a Friday night I would be met with refusals. Because meditation is not a recognised form of adrenalin-filled excitement, these refusals would not be deemed rude. But when the refusal is followed by an offer of a social dinner at their house the weekend after, I am expected to say yes or be deemed rude and miserable!

I think it should be a rule now that for every hour that you would like me to make polite conversation with you about your children or your career you should engage in an hour's meditation with me. In this way we can equally share each other's sources of personal fulfilment and grow together…

Now, the reason I am writing about this is not really to have some kind of a moan but rather to bring to people's attention something that I feel many practitioners of the internal arts also experience. I suspect that some of you reading this recognise some of these issues and perhaps even feel the same. I find these issues kind of funny, but I have met internal practitioners for whom this has become a major problem in their lives. The discomfort with these kinds of social gatherings leads to a kind of experiential pressure that can turn into feelings of depression and inadequacy. Projected views of being miserable and unsociable are transferred onto them by outside people and this then creates an actual reality.

I have even met some who misunderstood what was going on in their development and so instead used their 'unsociability' as a sign of internal progress – 'I have trained meditation for so long that I am now incapable of mixing with other people.' This becomes a form of unconscious arrogance as they place themselves above those who are able to socialise. Perhaps this is because unsociability is equated with reaching the stage of becoming a hermit practitioner?

The truth is that even though I have difficulty with social events and other projected forms of fun, I still have to do it. I recognise that I am in the minority and it is also an important skill to learn how to blend and mix with others. If I had to give one practical reason why this is the case it is simply because mindset and energy are projected between people very easily. If many people in your social network perceive you as unsocial and miserable then this negative energy gradually becomes attached to you and essentially this is negative for your cultivation. It is better to be liked by those around you. There is no benefit to being disliked; this adds to the difficulties cultivating your internal energy. If this means joining in with others' socially accepted forms of fun then that is fine – it is a small price to pay. If I could not even put up with a social evening making small talk because it made me feel unhappy then I have really achieved very little. Feelings like boredom are things that need to be tackled and shed just like any other negative feelings or emotions. I also find that since I have no major wish to share details about my life through small talk with those around me I am happy just to sit and listen to people at social gatherings. For many this can be quite powerful, and I see that in some cases it has served as a form of effective transformative therapy for them. Most conversations involve a lot of talking and very little listening. If you can inject a little more listening into a social event then you have the power really to help somebody touch the part of their being that can change for the better. I see this as a service that more people should give and an extension of the skills of my study.

If I stick to this way of thinking then even an awkward social event that I ultimately find detracts from my valuable training time can become a form of alchemical practice. For those of you experiencing the same difficulties in your own lives perhaps you could try viewing it in the same way? Even if we will never get the majority of our friends to join us for meditation the weekend after!

16

TRANSCRIBED LECTURE ON ALCHEMY

Damo Mitchell

Qi Gong comes from within the umbrella practice of Nei Gong, which is the process of internal transformation inherent within such exercises. Even deeper than Nei Gong is the practice of Nei Dan Gong. Often translated as 'internal alchemy', Nei Dan Gong actually translates as the 'internal elixir skill'.

Most who come into contact with Daoism begin their training through exercises such as Qi Gong. Qi Gong, as most people know, is a slow-moving form of health-preservation exercise based around linking the body, the breath and the mind into a single unit. Through consistent practice a person is able to increase their health, calm their mind, increase the flow of vital energy around their body and also gain a window into the more complicated and wider picture of the Daoist tradition.

In understanding the word 'skill', we have to look at the Chinese term 'Gong' (功). People think when they practise Qi Gong that they are actually practising Qi Gong. In fact, they are not. They are practising the exercises that would lead them towards Qi Gong and lead them towards the state of gaining the skill of controlling their energy. Only someone who has mastered the internal practices of Daoism will have achieved Qi Gong. We are working towards this. The same goes for Nei Gong. Those who manage to master the art of working with the various facets of their inner self will be said to have achieved Nei Gong, the skill of controlling the inner transformation process. In this respect, Nei Dan Gong is the same.

Internal alchemists, through consistent practice, will gain the skill of achieving the internal elixir, the Dan. The Dan is that which is sought out through the diligent practice of internal alchemy in order to create a substance that a person can then absorb and transfer throughout the body in order to lead them towards elevated states of consciousness and ultimately, according to the ancient tradition of Daoism, immortality. Oftentimes people call Nei Dan Gong, or internal alchemy, Daoist meditation – which is true – but in fact we must look and try to understand what meditation actually is in order to find out if internal alchemy fits into one of these categories. In general, most forms of meditation can be divided into five main categories.

The first is visualisation. Meditations based around visualisation generally involve the person sitting, closing their eyes, breathing and trying to create an image within their head. This may be the picture of a flower, a light, a colour or a movement through the body, etc. Sometimes it involves constructing a complex mental image in the form of a mandala or a sacred place that they choose to visit through their mind's eye. Visualisation, essentially, is an external form of meditation because it is based around the use of the mind, rather than the use of true consciousness or any form of mental stillness.

The second form of meditation is contemplative practice. This, in my opinion, is not really meditation. Contemplation is more akin to a state of deep thinking, wherein the person tries to enter into a state of relative quietude and then see beyond the external layers of their acquired mind to try and find an answer to something that has been confusing them or troubling them for some time. Contemplation is a tool used by meditation practitioners, but some would argue that perhaps the answers they're seeking should come automatically out of the stillness found within other forms of meditation, rather than through contemplation.

The third system of meditation is devotion, or religious meditation, wherein the practitioner often visualises a deity or a sacred spirit that is important to them and usually relevant to the religion they practise. From here they attempt to gain a connection through that devotional meditation to this spiritual deity. Prayer is a form of devotional meditation.

The fourth form of meditation is emptiness. Many forms of meditation often fit into this, whereby a person aims to simply achieve true stillness in their mind – to think about nothing. Perhaps they follow their breath as a way to enter into their state and essentially allow the ego, or the acquired mind, to dissolve of its own accord.

The fifth and final form of meditation is alchemical, sometimes known as Tantric, which involves taking various subtle energies within the body and working with them to create a change of state or a change of consciousness. Nei Gong, Daoist internal alchemy, is a form of alchemical meditation.

Daoist internal alchemy is the core of the entire tradition of Daoism. Many of the realisations that generated Daoist art came from internal alchemy, such as Chinese medicine, martial arts, astronomy, astrology, etc. If we look at the theory of Daoist internal alchemy it can seem very complex at first. This is in part due to the complexities of working with the internal environment of the body and also the fact that so much of it was written about in metaphorical language.

Daoist Nei Dan has a very comprehensive set of guidelines, structures and theoretical concepts that inform the practice. If we shrink this down slightly, we get Nei Gong theory, and if we shrink it down even more, what we get is Qi Gong theory. So, if you're encountering Daoist internal alchemy for the first time, you'll find that you are already familiar with a lot of the terms and a lot of the practices, but perhaps it will go a little bit deeper than you are used to if you've only studied something like Qi Gong before.

Many people who have encountered other forms of meditation will find that right from the beginning they're told to sit, fold their legs, close their eyes and settle the mind. Now, for the occasional few, that can be a life-changing experience and they can touch upon heightened states of consciousness and elevated levels of awareness. But for the vast majority, it becomes an impossible task.

Alchemy realises this difficulty and places steps before the stages of entering emptiness. So prior to sitting and forgetting, the person has to work with various base frequencies and energies within their body so that what they have is a step-by-step process in order to lead them into this state. It is only when they've gone through these various stages of transformation, and they have been led into the stage of sitting and forgetting, that they begin to attain union with a higher state of consciousness, generally referred to as Dao within Daoism.

Two important terms to become familiar with, if you are studying alchemy, are Xian Tian and Hou Tian, or pre-Heaven and post-Heaven. I tend to translate these as congenital and acquired. That which is congenital, the Xian Tian, comes before birth – literally, before existence. In Daoist theory, cosmology, your consciousness, is given to you from heaven. Your spirit, your life, is lent to you by the heavens, along with your soul, until such a time when you die. Anything that comes from this state is congenital, Xian Tian. Xian Tian can only be contacted when we are in the state of true inner stillness.

The acquired, the Hou Tian, is that which comes after your birth. With regards to your mind, the congenital is your true state of being – the stillness at the centre of your consciousness that we are trying to contact through the practice of meditation. The acquired are the layers of mind that build up over the course of your life through things you've learned, things you've experienced, biases, interactions with others and so on. The problem is that most people identify solely with the acquired nature and not enough with the congenital. We require both, but essentially we must be able to see through the mire of the acquired mind so that the congenital can see through to the outside world. In studying this we need to understand the difference between stillness and movement. Daoism tells us that the congenital is based around stillness. As soon as something moves, it transforms from stillness to movement. It transforms from congenital to acquired.

In understanding this, we need to understand the theory of Yin and Yang, and the balance between stillness and movement. If we can master both of these things, then we are able to – as Daoists say – return to the source. When we return to the source, an undistorted state of consciousness can be born. It is at this stage that we are said to have entered into the state of being a sage.

The model that Daoists use for understanding the internal universe of the human body is entitled 'the three treasures'. These are Jing, Qi and Shen. Jing is often translated as our 'essence', Qi is often translated as our 'energy' and Shen is generally translated as our 'spirit'. If you were to study Qi Gong theory in Chinese medicine you would be very, very familiar with these terms. For internal alchemy, we need to go a little bit deeper. Jing can be divided into the congenital and the acquired. The Yuan Jing, the original essence, is the congenital. It is the vibratory pattern that contains the potential for existence. When Jing then moves from the congenital to the acquired, your essence transforms via the action of movement. From here, it starts to create life processes as well as fluids within the body, in particular your sexual essences.

Qi, your energy, can also be divided into congenital and acquired. Congenital Qi, sometimes known as the original energy or sometimes the original breath, Yuan Xi, is that which is gifted to you from the movement of original spirit. When it begins to circulate through the body, it becomes the acquired Qi – the acquired energy. The acquired energy is formed from the food that we eat and the air that we breathe as they mix within the body and circulate through the meridian system; the acquired Qi is that which gives us life.

Your spirit is the Shen. When Shen is in a congenital state it is a pure white light of enlightenment that most people who reach elevated states of consciousness will experience glowing inside the mind's eye. When it enters the state of Hou Tian, the acquired state, your spirit refracts into parts. These go on to interact with each other to give us our state of consciousness, and when they're out of balance they produce emotional imbalances and emotional shifts that give us the formation of the acquired mind.

These three are linked because, though essentially they are three, they are one. Your Jing can change into Qi if it is raised in vibration. It can be converted into Shen – spirit – if it is raised higher. In the same way, if your spirit is slowed it becomes your energy. And your energy, if slowed, becomes your essence. Figure 16.1 shows the movements and conversion of the three treasures.

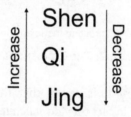

FIGURE 16.1: THE CONVERSIONS OF JING, QI AND SHEN

Internally, the movement of your energy takes place through the Jing Luo (经络), the meridian system. The meridian system, or the energy body, is divided into various parts. But for simplicity it is easier to understand the alchemical language of the eight congenital channels and the 12 acquired channels. Daoism discusses that the 12 acquired – or organ – channels are that which circulate energy after you are born. These are the meridians you will often see written about within acupuncture books or shiatsu texts. When we are practising simple Qi Gong exercises we are generally circulating energy within these 12 channels.

At the centre, deeper within the body, are the eight congenital meridians. The eight congenital meridians form a network, a cage-shaped set of circuits that surround the three Dan Tien, as shown in Figure 16.2.

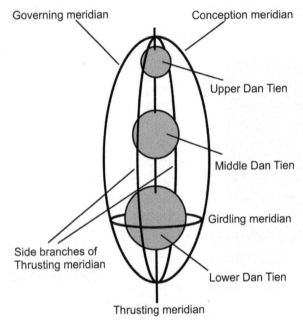

FIGURE 16.2: THE CONGENITAL CAGE

Within Qi Gong theory it is stated that these channels serve as reservoirs of energy, but in fact they do much more than this. Alchemy is based around creating movement within these channels and creating expansion in order to generate heat inside so that any conversions within the body take place within these eight extraordinary meridians. As well as this, we have something that Daoists simply term the 'ten thousand collaterals' within our body. Whenever you see the number 'ten thousand' in Chinese terminology, especially in classical texts, it generally just means a large number. You could equate it with infinity. The ten thousand collaterals are small branches that run off the other meridians within the energy body connecting the skin, the tissue, the bones and the organs into one unit. If you were able to see these pathways it would look something like a large mass of wool tangled up throughout the body. It would be impossible to map them out accurately.

In the early stages of alchemy we are aiming to move energy through the 12 organ channels and the ten thousand collaterals. As we become better at our practice and move deeper into alchemy, it is the eight congenital meridians that we seek to open up and create movement within. Controlling and opening these channels gives us a space to carry out our alchemical practice. If alchemy can be equated to the formation of rare metals from base substances – the conversion of lead to gold – we can also equate our body to being something like a workshop. If our workshop is a mess, we won't produce good results. The concept of Daoist internal alchemy is that we open the channels within the body – the ten thousand collaterals – to create an effective workshop within which we can carry out our alchemy. Although, in this case, we're not converting lead to gold – we're converting acquired spirit to original nature. This process is summarised in Figure 16.3.

Prepare the body
↓
Open the key meridians
↓
Open the 'ten thousand collaterals'
↓
Consolidate the Jing
↓
Regulate the Qi
↓
Still the acquired mind
↓
Locate the congenital nature
↓
Cultivate the true spirit

FIGURE 16.3: ALCHEMICAL CONVERSION

In order to do this, we need to find the various sources of movement and conversion within our body and return them to the stillness of potential. This is called returning to Dao or converting spirit to emptiness. In the early stages, we must understand that we can only work in a certain order. You cannot work with your energy system until you have worked with your body. You cannot work with your spirit until you have worked with your energy system. The body must be the root of everything you do. Our physicality is gifted to us through our essence, through our Jing. The quality of our Jing dictates the health of our physical form. For this reason, Daoists talk about the preservation of essence, or Jing, in the early stages.

The study of the preservation of Jing and the conversion of your physical health into a high enough state to practise alchemy is called Yang Sheng (养身). Literally translated, Yang Sheng means life nourishing or healthy living. It is important to understand that Jing is the base frequency that gives birth to both our sexual fluids and emotional states such as desire. The Daoist theory of consciousness states that spirit is rooted in physicality. If you wish to picture it as something more tangible you could think of your spirit as being like a balloon filled with helium tied to a weight that stops it floating back to the heavens. That weight is the physical form of your body. When you die this string is cut, and thus the root of your spirit is severed, as shown in Figure 16.4.

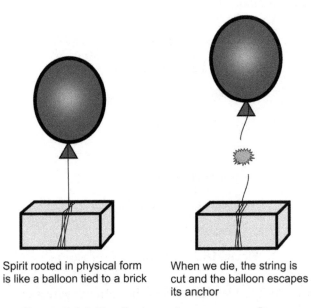

Spirit rooted in physical form
is like a balloon tied to a brick

When we die, the string is
cut and the balloon escapes
its anchor

FIGURE 16.4: THE PHYSICAL ANCHORING OF SPIRIT

Every aspect of your physical body has an aspect of consciousness linked to it. For example, your anger and the associated emotional traits of your character are linked to the Liver. Excitation is linked to your Heart, grief is linked to your Lungs and fear to your Kidneys. Your sexual desire is linked to your essence and your sexual fluids. In this way spirit, physicality and emotional traits are intertwined. Excessive sexual activity in Daoism would be against healthy, life-nourishing principles. Sexual desire is obviously that which causes you to use up your sexual fluids. Daoism looks at consolidating the Jing, storing the essence and going against your sexual desire in the early stages of practice, particularly for men. Within the West, we say that people's sex lives worsen as they become older. Daoism takes the opposite view; it says the more you have sex, the more your age increases. So, a person who does not guard their essence and gives in constantly to their sexual desire will age and weaken a lot faster than somebody who understands how to cultivate and recirculate their essence.

Remember though that in Daoism we are not aiming to age the physical body backwards. It would not be wise or possible for us to do this. We cannot return to being a toddler and then a baby. Rather, we aim to slow down the ageing process and then work backwards energetically. When you are born your energy system is in a certain state; as you become an adult it transforms. As you become elderly it is transformed into something else. We cannot return backwards along this ageing process but we can reverse the process of ageing energetically inside of our body. This is the conversion of movement to stillness that forms the basis for all alchemical practices.

A bonus effect of this is an increase in health and longevity. But remember that this was never the aim of Daoism. Daoism's aim was transcendent comprehension and, by the time it became alchemy, immortality. At no point was it ever the study of longevity. This just came as a by-product of the alchemical practices that they were exploring. Within Daoism the term Xing means nature. Your nature is very, very important. In understanding our nature, we must understand the nature of mind and we must understand the nature of consciousness. When the two interact with each other adequately then the virtuous side of your nature will come out and true nature or Xing will have been achieved.

The second term to become familiar with is Ming. Ming is often translated as destiny by many scholars of Chinese theory, but actually its meaning goes a lot deeper. Ming can be better understood as your life path. It is the route that you take from your birth to your death and everything that happens to you along the way, so a person who has had a very bumpy Ming will be someone who is said to have had lots of difficulties during their life, maybe lots of illnesses and lots of catastrophes or obstacles to overcome. Someone with a steady Ming will be someone who has moved very smoothly and easily from birth to death with good health and a high level of longevity. Our Ming also dictates the level of our awareness of the Will of Heaven.

The Will of Heaven is more akin to your destiny because it is that which is laid down to you by the heavens. Essentially, when esoteric Daoists talk about Heaven, what they mean is the movement of the planets, the stars and the constellations. This is the reason for the importance of astrology and astronomy within Daoism. Religious Daoism talks about the Will of Heaven actually being an intervention by deities and gods within a person's life, but alchemy is essentially a form of esoteric Daoism rather than a religious practice.

Your Ming is also your health. The reason the Ming is your health is that your body is the vehicle that you use in order to move along your life path. If your body is unhealthy, if your body is sick, then it is like trying to travel down a road in a poor vehicle. We cannot ignore our physical health if we are to engage in any esoteric practices because we must have all of our spirits and energies rooted in something strong. If we understand this, and these different meanings for Ming, we can see why it's difficult to translate that term literally. In understanding Ming in this way you can see how your physical health, your fate and your path through life is interchangeably woven into one unit. Through working with Ming we must work with our physical body and our path through life as well as our preordained reason for existence. If we can convert this, then we'll start to change our Xing.

In understanding the basis of meditation or alchemical theory within Daoism, we can see that Daoists are trying to work on a combination of Xing and Ming. Only when Xing and Ming come together will a person be able to achieve Nei Dan Gong – the skill of locating the inner elixir. Many forms of meditation focus on Xing to the exclusion of Ming. This means they are only working on the mental level. People who practise only Xing-based systems may be happy and they may be calm, but they generally have poor posture, weak muscles and poor health. They do not live too long. They have cultivated nature completely to the exclusion of worrying about their body.

Many Daoist practitioners do the opposite. They focus on Ming to the exclusion of Xing. They're working on their physical health to the exclusion of their nature. People who practise in this manner will practise life-nourishing techniques such as medical Qi Gong or

Taijiquan for health. They'll do anything they can to increase their Qi flow, guard their essence and make sure they're healthy, but they will completely ignore the cultivation of mind. This is considered an imbalanced method. If a person does not work their Xing – their nature – as well as working with their body, they may reach states of great internal attainment, but they will not have the refined understanding of ethics to go alongside it. A person like this is dangerous. They may develop superhuman abilities on certain levels but they will not understand the wrong and right way to use these abilities.

If we want to achieve true transcendence – or what the Daoists call the state of a Xian, an immortal – we must cultivate Xing and Ming evenly and bring them together. If we picture our nature – Xing – and our life path – Ming – as two opposite poles, the chain links that connect these two together are Jing, Qi and Shen: our essence, our energy and our spirit. By working with these three we work with the chain links to pull our Xing and Ming in line with each other. When the two come together, that is the way to master the skill of Nei Dan Gong.

17

SPINAL FIRES
Part 1
Damo Mitchell

This chapter looks at one aspect of the Daoist Tantric traditions. It is actually an aspect of internal training that I studied within a slightly unusual Daoist line. It is quite separate from the alchemical or philosophical traditions. For me it is always fascinating to see just how many different ways the teachings of Daoism were interpreted and expressed around Asia.

Entering the deeper aspects of Daoist internal work can be intimidating. Instructions are often shrouded in metaphorical language and teachings can appear contradictory. It can take a number of years to even begin to grasp what is supposed to take place within the body, and this often relies on having access to the correct teachers and the correct methods. Trying to achieve this understanding has been a large part of my own exploration throughout the years. My understanding of the human energy system, as it stands now, is the result of a thorough exploration of different esoteric schools (primarily within the Daoist tradition), combined with my own personal experience. Once much of the metaphorical language is stripped away, you are left with a fairly simple model of the human mind/body system, which can be systematically worked through using various internal methods. These methods can be seen in different forms of Qi Gong, Nei Gong and alchemy as well as within some branches of the older internal martial arts systems. Classical texts and charts such as the Nei Jing Tu (內经图), the Xiuzhen Tu (修真图) and the Cantong Qi (參同契) elaborate on these methods. In order to understand these methods, you must be able to decode the language used by the ancient Daoists.

Specific exercises, such as ancient Dao Yin, contain direct methods for preparing the body for higher-level spiritual work – providing the practitioner can understand exactly how to approach the exercises. Many of the more complex aspects of Daoist internal work can be accessed through specific exercises that serve to provide a solid foundation for the more complicated study of Daoist meditation practice.

The spine, along with its associated energetic properties, constitutes one of the most important aspects of the human body. It is said that if a person can take care of their spine, the rest of their body will be healthy. The spinal cord is the 'pillar' that extends between Heaven and Earth. As a teacher, I have consistently found that work with the spine is what many internal artists lack; genuine skill can be developed very quickly by manipulating the spine correctly.

In order to understand the function of the spine with regards to the higher levels of Daoist internal work, we must first look at the various branches of the meridian system that run through this area of the body.

- The first energetic branch of the meridian system that runs through the area of the back is the Du or 'governing' meridian. This is the most Yang of the congenital meridians. Originating at the sacrum, it runs up the centre of the back. It then runs over the top of the head and ends right underneath the nose. This meridian governs the Yang functions of the body and circulates Qi into the Yang-organ meridians of the body throughout the course of our daily lives. It is paired with the Ren or 'conception' meridian, which continues this circulation of Qi down the front of the body, under the perineum and back into the Du meridian. The Ren meridian governs the Yin functions of the body and directs Qi into all the Yin-organ meridians of the body. Together, they form a loop of circulating energy, which helps to regulate the entire energy body and divide the two poles of Yin and Yang. When beginning any form of Daoist internal work, it is crucial to set up a good circulation through these two channels. This circulation is often known as the 'small water wheel of Qi' or the 'microcosmic orbit'. The early stages of many systems of Qi Gong and Nei Gong work towards establishing this circulation of Qi within the body.

- The next energetic branch to be aware of is the central branch of the Chong Mai. Once the Qi is effectively circulating within the Du and Ren orbits, as described above, it is then possible for movement to begin taking place along the length of the central branch of the Chong Mai. This surge of energy starts at the base of the body around the area of the perineum and moves up towards the crown of the head through the body's core. This movement of energy causes Jing to be converted into Qi and Qi into Shen as the refining functions of the three Dan Tien are awakened. This helps to nourish the upper Dan Tien and brain with spiritual energy. It also sets up a kind of 'spiritual antenna' in the Chong Mai, which helps to connect a person to divine information drawn directly from Dao.

- The third branch of the energy system directly connected with this area of the body – and the spine in particular – is the spinal branch of the Chong Mai. Some of the more advanced stages of Nei Gong and Nei Dan training rely on creating a strong movement of Qi along this channel. The spinal branch of the Chong Mai and the Du meridian are not the same thing though. They are different channels with different functions (see Figure 17.1). This causes a great deal of confusion for many practitioners of the internal arts. However, understanding the difference between these two pathways is quite simple. We only have to look at the nature of what moves through each of these channels.

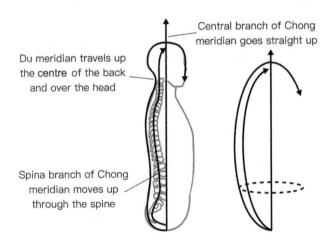

FIGURE 17.1: THE DU AND CHONG MERIDIANS

Movement along the central branch of the Chong Mai takes place as Jing converts into Qi and Qi into Shen. This begins the process of sending extra spiritual energy towards the upper Dan Tien, which can bring experiences of connection with Dao and divine insights. These experiences can be brief at first but, with practice, it is possible to remain for longer periods of time in a state of union with Dao.

Deeper spine work engages the spiritual aspect of this part of our body. In order to do this, we must activate specific areas of the spine, referred to as the 'seven spinal fires'. These seven points govern the movement from our congenital nature into the acquired. Remnants of these theories can be seen in modern Chinese medical practices, which still refer to one of the spiritual fires, known as Ming Men. Ming Men is now known as the expansion of energy that takes place around the area of the Kidneys. However, it was originally seen as one of seven spiritual fires that dictate our acquired connection to Ming – our predetermined path through life. These seven spiritual fires are often depicted as seven (or sometimes nine in other traditions) cauldrons that are located along the length of the spine, as shown in Figure 17.2.

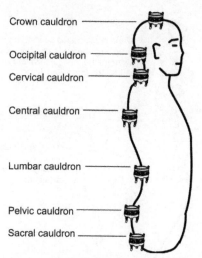

Crown cauldron

Occipital cauldron

Cervical cauldron

Central cauldron

Lumbar cauldron

Pelvic cauldron

Sacral cauldron

FIGURE 17.2: THE SPINAL CAULDRONS

In order to work with these seven spiritual fires, we must first have a strong flow of Qi along the length of the spinal branch of the Chong Mai. Once the spinal pathway is clear, it is possible to work with the spinal fires.

The spinal fires are the Daoist tradition's equivalent of the Chakra in Yoga. Whether you refer to them as Chakra or spinal fires, you must make sure to distinguish them from the three Dan Tien, as they are quite separate from the circulation of Qi taking place within the Du and the Ren. In fact, they exist on completely different levels of frequency. The three Dan Tien, and anything related to the flow of Qi through the meridian system, exist within the realm of the energy body. By contrast, the spinal fires exist within the realm of the spirit/consciousness body. Understanding this distinction helps us to monitor our personal progress through our training. Figure 17.3 shows the different frequencies that determine the level of existence of each of these aspects of our inner universe.

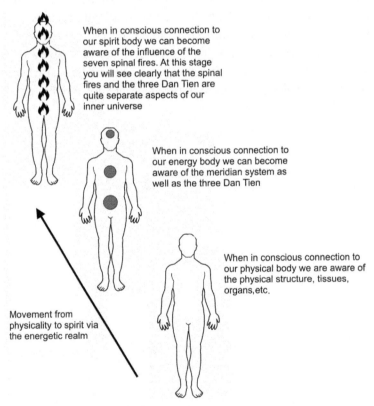

When in conscious connection to our spirit body we can become aware of the influence of the seven spinal fires. At this stage you will see clearly that the spinal fires and the three Dan Tien are quite separate aspects of our inner universe

When in conscious connection to our energy body we can become aware of the meridian system as well as the three Dan Tien

When in conscious connection to our physical body we are aware of the physical structure, tissues, organs, etc.

Movement from physicality to spirit via the energetic realm

FIGURE 17.3: COMPARATIVE FREQUENCIES

As shown above, each of these different elements exists within one of the three human bodies.

Whether we can access a certain level of frequency (and its associated aspects) depends on what stage we have reached in our practice. In the early days, we are generally connected solely to the physical realm, governed by our five senses. As we progress through an art such as Qi Gong, we can begin to 'tune' into the energy body and feel the flow of Qi and the rotation of the Dan Tien. Only when this has been worked through can we go further and connect with the spirit body, which exists at a much higher range of frequency. Our ability to connect with our true consciousness depends on our ability to reach into the realm of spiritual energy (Shen). In order to achieve this stage, we must have refined our internal sensitivity to a high level. The spirit body can only be accessed through periods of profound inner stillness. This is where the energy of the spine comes into play.

According to Daoist thought, the extreme emptiness of Wuji is the point where human consciousness originates. This spark of original intention is known as our 'seed consciousness'; it is the aspect of our consciousness that carries the divine information, giving us the potential for spiritual liberation within our current lifetime. Our congenital nature is the manifestation of true human consciousness, born forth from the seed consciousness. It is this aspect of consciousness that manifests the sage-like compassionate qualities of the De, which we would manifest if we were able to free ourselves from the shackles of mind. Emotions govern the majority of our thoughts, speech and actions. Emotions move like waves out of our congenital nature – by nature, they are constantly shifting. By distorting our thoughts, emotions prevent us from successfully tapping into our own congenital nature. These emotional cognitive distortions give birth to our acquired nature, which builds up over the course of our lives, layer upon layer. Our acquired nature is the aspect of our mind that is governed by logic, bias and prejudice. In new-age thought, the acquired mind is usually referred to as the 'ego' – the aspect of human self that we falsely identify with. The acquired mind is mapped out in Figure 17.4.

In its stages of development, consciousness can be seen as moving outwards in concentric circles. Through a spiritual form of centrifugal movement, the stillness of our true self expands to create our congenital nature first and then our acquired nature. The deeper aspects of Daoist training aim at working with the layers of our acquired nature. We use our acquired nature to navigate our everyday lives, and it is also through the distorted lens of our acquired nature that we view the nature of the world. The Daoist tradition was concerned with shedding the layers of the acquired nature in order to revert back to the congenital aspect of our consciousness. In theory, this should allow us to contact the stillness directly that exists at the heart of everything. By moving beyond any form of individual identification, we come in direct union with Dao. Every aspect of Daoist philosophy has a direct, literal counterpart in the microcosm of the human organism that can be experienced through our practice. The nature of the human mind is no exception to this. Upon touching the stillness that sits at our very core, we should understand how our own consciousness formed from this point and begin to dissolve the layers of acquired nature that have been building up throughout our lives.

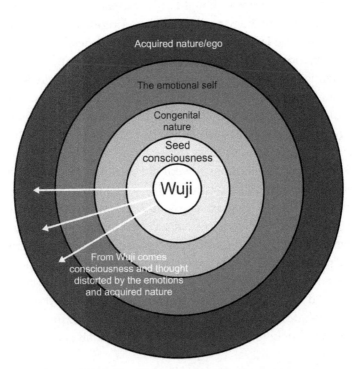

FIGURE 17.4: THE LAYERS OF HUMAN CONSCIOUSNESS

Practices such as Nei Gong or internal alchemy allow us to raise Jing, Qi and Shen through the central branch of the Chong Mai. This gradually enables us to bring the three bodies together into one unified whole. The more we are able to do this, the more likely it is that the 'mysterious pass' can begin to open up for us. As this pass opens, it gives us a direct connection to Dao, which helps to dissolve the layers of the acquired nature that have built up. The more we practise, the longer we are able to remain within this state and lead our minds towards stillness. The spinal branch of the Chong Mai contains stillness at its core. This branch serves as a conduit for our own consciousness, energy system and physical form to move through. This is the reason why it is such a powerful aspect of the energy body when we are working on our own internal development.

There are several expanding areas of information along the length of the spine. Those centres help to 'step down' the frequency of Dao into consciousness. When you connect with these seven fires, it feels as though they are vibrating and spiralling at the same time. The spinal fires are smaller than the three Dan Tien – they are roughly a centimetre in diameter. Each of these spinal fires is connected to a different aspect of our consciousness and how it develops; as they open up, a major shift in our perception takes place. Figure 17.5 shows the location of the seven spinal fires.

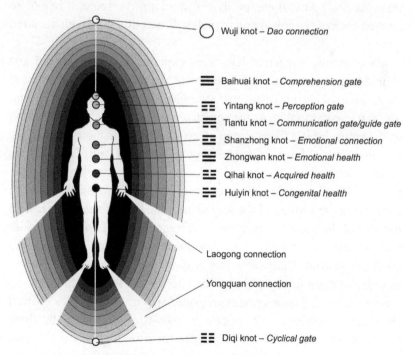

FIGURE 17.5: THE SPINAL FIRES

As shown in Figure 17.5, each of these fires is directly connected to a different layer or our energy field, which stores information throughout the course of our lives. As we move deep into our practice and awaken each of the spinal fires, any negative information associated with a particular fire begins to dissolve. This loss of accumulated information then enables true consciousness to move from our core into our external being, causing a major shift of perception. The stronger we can make these shifts in perception, the more we are able to stabilise our mind. Stabilising our mind not only changes the way we relate to the outside world but also enables us to refine our energy into spirit within the central branch of our Chong Mai in a more efficient way.

The more we can open up the energetic pathway within the spine, the more we are able to direct spiritual information up through the spiritual fires. At first we will only be shifting Qi through our spine, resulting in the spontaneous reactions associated with this stage of development. However, after a while, we will begin to lift a more refined energy along the length of the spine and up into the centre of the brain, at a point known as the 'mud pill palace' within alchemical texts. As this spiritual energy moves up along the spine, it begins to awaken each of the spinal fires, which will start dissolving our acquired nature.

It is usually expected that every experience in the internal arts should be pleasant. This is definitely not the case, in my experience at least. Some of the processes that take place in the body and the mind are very uncomfortable. As the spiritual energy moves along the length of the spine, it feels like a strong electric current passing through you. It comes with a sharp, 'electrical' type of pain that causes the muscles to contract and relax spasmodically, as if you were plugged into a powerful TENS machine. These electrical shocks move quickly through the centre of the spine, all the way up into the base of the neck, around the area of the occiput. They then discharge into the base of your skull with a great deal of power. The first time I experienced this, I actually cried out in pain. Classically, this is supposed to happen three times in order to open up the point at the base of the skull – although, on a personal level, I have only experienced two of these shocks. Within alchemical traditions, this process is known as 'receiving the three strikes of thunder', and it serves to open the strongly blocked point on the base of your skull, known in many traditions as the 'jade pillow' or, more appropriately, the 'thunder-strike centre'. Once the point at the base of the skull has been opened, the spiritual energy surges right up into the centre of your brain. When it reaches this point, the electric shock strikes the 'mud pill palace', resulting in a strong electrical shock. This feels even worse than the pain involved in the first part of the process! When I experienced it, the shock caused me to pass out. The first time it happened, I was meditating with a group of around 25 people – which was rather embarrassing!

When I first started writing, I originally decided not to include any practices that involved any danger. I did not want to share information that could cause harm. There is often fear around certain practices in the internal arts. After writing my first book, I received many messages from people around the world who had experienced some of the stages I described in the book on their own. Some of these people had trained in similar systems, while others had simply stumbled on the process without really knowing what they were doing. The vast majority of people had acknowledged the experience with a degree of curiosity and carried on with their training. A few others had suffered quite severe health problems that they could not easily receive help with. The fact is that many internal practices come with a certain degree of risk, if they are not practised correctly and under the guidance of an experienced teacher. In the case of simple Qi Gong exercises, these risks are almost non-existent. However, once you start going deeper into the internal arts, you are essentially beginning to work with the various elements that make up your nature. Many people are starting to move into these stages anyway, so I figured I might as well include them in my writings so that the information is available.

First, let us be clear on one thing. In order to reach the stage of activating the spinal fires, you must have trained for *a long time*. This is not something that will happen to you within the first few years of your training; beginners need not worry. In order for this process to begin, the spinal branch of the Chong Mai must be fully open – and this is no mean feat. It took me many years to do this, and I have the luxury of not having any major commitments in my life other than my practice and my school. I have been a full-time practitioner now for many years, and even with the amount of hours I am able to put into my practice, it still took a long time to even begin to touch on this stage. You must already have a fully awakened energy system, the lower Dan Tien should be rotating smoothly and the majority of the Qi Men (氣門) (energy gates) points throughout your body need to be open. Those not prepared to put in hours of daily practice are unlikely ever to reach this stage, but I have included it here for those who do put this amount of time into their training.

There are various techniques for raising the spiritual energy towards the spinal fires, but it generally happens as a by-product of other alchemical work. The spiritual energy will move of its own accord when it is ready.

If it is ready then it will move very quickly up along the length of your spine towards the 'thunder-strike centre' point at the base of your skull. If this happens, simply relax and allow it to do what it wants. You may experience the first of three shocks at the base of your skull. In my own experience, these shocks were separated by a couple of years. It took about five years between the first shock at the base of my skull and the second one at the centre of my brain. Most of the time, this energy did not want to rise up. In the Hindu tradition, this rising energy is referred to as the Kundalini; it is said to coil like two snakes along the length of the spine. Because of these teachings, I was expecting more of a coiling energy, rather than an electrical shock. But I was mistaken. I am not sure whether this means that the sensation is specific to each individual or if the Yogic method causes the spiritual energy to rise in a different manner. Unfortunately, this is not a question I can answer since I only have a rudimentary knowledge of higher-level Yogic practice. The only thing I know for certain is that the slightly unpleasant nature of this spiritual energy rising is also discussed within Yogic teachings.

As the energy rises along the length of the spine, it begins the process of awakening the seven fires. This is a gradual process that unfolds over a long period of time. Much like flowers blossoming open, those fires gradually begin to dissolve various aspects of the acquired mind. This causes various shifts in your consciousness. The fires start to awaken from the base of the spine upward – although this linear fashion only seems to apply about 90 per cent of the time. Occasionally, I get the feeling that different fires are active at different times. Once this process has begun, it is fuelled by your regular internal practices, especially sitting practice.

18

SPINAL FIRES
Part 2
Damo Mitchell

This chapter discusses the nature of each of the seven fires/ cauldrons, drawn from my own personal experience. Please be aware though that this is a very subjective account and your own experience may differ from mine. I have included my own experiences as a reference point to assist anybody going through the same process. I named each fire after key meridian points that exist in the same location. These are not their classical names – I have included the classical names in the descriptive text for each of the seven fires.

- **Sacral fire:** The first of the fires is the sacral fire, which is classically known as 'gateway to the tail'. The movement of spiritual energy along the base of the spine can feel very hot – almost as if your coccyx is burning. This experience only lasts for a short time, as the fire starts to awaken. As this area opens up, it can cause the entire body to shake violently from side to side. Extreme heat starts moving through the muscles and you will most likely be drenched in sweat as this happens.

  The sacral fire governs the 'base' aspects of your acquired nature. All of the key elements in life that you currently hold to be important are brought into question as this fire begins to awaken. These are usually to do with the beliefs given to you by your parents and other family members as you were growing up. Things like having a good career, owning a large house and being successful are considered to be important goals in life. Ideas about how you should fit into society and constantly seek to acquire new possessions were given to you by other people. Of course, none of these ideas are required to be happy and fulfilled in life. As the sacral fire begins to awaken, it is normal to start realising how ridiculous these ideas are. Throughout the process of awakening, you will naturally seek to make your life increasingly simple in order to focus on what is really important to you.

- **Ming Men fire:** Ming Men (命門) fire is classically known as the 'Ming fire' and is situated in the lower spine area, beneath the second lumbar vertebrae. As the spiritual energy begins to awaken this point, the heat increases and moves into the back. There is a lot more shaking and sweating as this point is reached! Again, this only lasts for a short time, as the awakening process begins.

  This fire is linked to your emotional programming. This concerns the lessons you received as you were growing up from people around you, society and the media – how you were taught to react to outside stimuli. Most people are not aware that their emotional reaction to the world is largely dictated by what they were taught at a young age. What makes you angry, sad, happy or stressed is often inherited from people around you. As this fire begins to awaken, it is normal for all of this to be brought into question. On a personal level, I found this to be quite a difficult process. As this spinal fire started to awaken, I went through an emotional meltdown – I was not able to deal with the outside world for a few months. Extreme paranoia hit me along with acute sensitivity to what everybody was feeling, especially if those feelings were directed towards me. This was very difficult but only temporary as my emotional nature received an overhaul. Afterwards, I had a much higher 'emotional threshold', meaning that it took a lot more for me to feel stressed, upset or angry. My emotions became a mere process I was able to observe, rather than something that governed my every thought. As an added bonus, my chronic digestive weakness (due to emotional stress) completely cleared up.

- **Zhong Shu fire:** Zhong Shu (中樞) fire is classically known as the 'earthen palace' and it is directly linked to your own sense of self. Its awakening comes with a great deal of energetic pressure in the centre of your body. This can cause you to throw your body backwards, thrusting your chest open towards the sky. If you are sitting down when this happens, it is quite normal to be thrown backwards onto the floor. As it opens, do not be surprised if you begin to cry or laugh hysterically as everything about your sense of self begins to fall away.

Everybody has an established perception of who we are. Usually, this is developed through our interactions with others and how they react to us. Over the course of our lives, we use other people as mirrors to understand who we are and how the rest of the world perceives us. This perception from those around us then dictates how we perceive ourselves; this is how we develop a warped sense of self. Most people never say what they are really thinking; thus, most information reflected back at us is a pure distortion. In this way, we create our own sense of self through our own dishonesty. When Zhong Shu fire begins to awaken, we can no longer lie to ourselves, as we see who we truly are. A deep realisation of our actual strengths, weaknesses and motives dawns on us, which means that we can begin to express a more honest version of who we are to others. This is a liberating stage, as people trying to maintain their false sense of self carry a great deal of tension.

- **Shen Dao fire:** Shen Dao (神道) fire is also known as the 'handle of the spine'. It is level with the heart and governs how we relate to others. As this fire awakens, it is normal to enter a state of bliss that can last for several months. During this time, it is as though you are walking around on 'cloud nine' with few cares in the world. The main drawback is that it becomes very difficult to carry out any tasks at work or at home, as they will be deemed completely irrelevant. You are truly carefree.

  As this fire awakens, your sense of true compassion is brought forth. The concept of hurting another seems like a completely mad idea, and a deep closeness with the rest of the world develops. For many people, this will be the first time that they will be able to experience unconditional love. This can change the way you relate to those around you in a deep way. Concepts such as sexism or racism will fade away, leaving you with the internal understanding that all human beings are equal across the planet. If everybody could open this spinal fire, the world would be a much more pleasant place.

- **Ya Men fire:** Ya Men (啞門) fire is known as the 'thunder-strike centre'. It sits at the base of the skull and is the point at which the spiritual energy first gets stuck when you are working at this level. Though the spiritual energy has moved through my spine past this point, I am only in the very early stages of awakening this fire. At the time of writing, I can only convey a very generic idea of what this point does, as I am sure I am only at a very basic level of attainment here. Ya Men fire governs our ability to communicate spiritually. As it awakens, you may start producing loud spontaneous sounds during your practice. You may end up chanting the 'ohm' sacred sound at the top of your voice for several hours – the 'ah' sound is another common sound that you may produce. Gradually, this may evolve into languages so ancient that you will not be able to translate them. This phenomenon, discussed in many spiritual traditions, lasts for a short time as Ya Men fire awakens.

  When this fire awakens, it is possible to speak from your true consciousness, without the filter of the acquired nature distorting your words in any way. When you speak to someone from this place, it bypasses their acquired nature. This will give a profound sense of truth to your words, which might resound deeply for whoever you're speaking to. I have only had glimpses of this when, occasionally, I have managed to speak from this deep place of inner stillness. Sadly, these have been fleeting moments of wisdom before returning to the clumsy public speaker I normally am! I have had teachers in the past who had fully awakened this fire, and everything they taught rung bells and opened doors within my heart and mind. Those who have fully awakened this gate should be the true internal teachers – people like myself are just amateurs in comparison.

- **Yin Tang fire:** Yin Tang (印堂) fire is also known as the 'bright hall'. It corresponds to the location of the third eye. As this point awakens, it feels as if somebody is drilling through the front of your skull and this usually feels quite painful.

While I have not awakened this fire yet, I have experienced the sensation when high-level teachers have been transmitting information directly from their mind into my own. This transmission of information travels through your third eye directly into the upper Dan Tien and often leaves you with a dull headache. This was the classical method used to pass on a full internal system, as many of the deeper aspects of the internal arts cannot be taught through demonstration or verbal instruction. Classically, it was said that you could never fully understand the internal arts until a great master had taught you in this way.

When speaking with those who have awakened this fire, it is clear to see that they have drawn divine understanding of their art and the nature of the cosmos from a place beyond the realm of human thought. They become like walking encyclopaedias of their tradition, with knowledge far beyond what can normally be learnt in one lifetime. It is as though they are being given the information directly from a higher source. I have only had the good fortune to meet a couple of teachers who had reached this stage and their teachings were life changing.

- **Bai Hui fire:** Bai Hui (百會) fire is also known as the 'crown fire'. I only had the chance to meet one teacher in Thailand who I believe had fully awakened this fire. This is the fire of connection to Wuji. While I have no idea what it feels like to awaken this fire, I know that the result must be extremely profound. The connection upwards to higher levels was so strong in this teacher that he took his students through the process of internal awakening just by allowing them to be around him. His very presence moved energy and shifted consciousness through my body without any verbal instruction being given. This is the way that true teachers passed on these arts, according to the legendary tales from traditions such as Daoism, Buddhism or Hinduism.

It is a curious aspect of the Daoist arts that the process of awakening the seven spinal fires is not actually required for those wishing to connect with Wuji and return their spirit to Dao. It is possible to go through this process by 'simply' using the refinement of Jing into Qi and Qi into Shen via the central branch of the Chong Mai. This is enough to create a direct connection with the divine and ultimately achieve what the ancient Daoists called immortality. For this reason, many systems of Daoism focus only on this process in their teachings. It is not even required to open the mysterious pass and bring forth the virtuous aspects of the De to be able to connect with Dao. This essentially means that the process is quite simple, if you want it to be this way. However, it comes with one great risk. If you do not need to bring forth the De or dissolve the acquired nature to reach high levels with your internal training, this means that you do not need to be a good person.

Many other spiritual traditions rely on external rules to tell students how to conduct themselves when they begin their spiritual training. Systems such as Buddhism have specific guidelines to ensure people interact with honesty and integrity. Daoism, on the other hand, has no such ethical structure. Sometimes a teacher may discuss ethical conduct, but it is certainly not given the priority in Daoism that it may have in other traditions. Daoism believes that any way you may choose to conduct yourself is false, unless it comes from deep within your true consciousness. Thus, only virtuous behaviour coming from the core of your congenital nature is considered virtuous. Any other reason for virtuous behaviour is false, as it is the result of external guidance. Whilst this ideal has its strengths, it also has its weaknesses. It is true that, at higher stages in the internal arts, you have the potential of developing certain abilities that are beyond most people. Abilities such as telepathy and similar skills are part of the internal arts and act as a sign that you are developing in the right direction. While these skills should never be the endgame of these practices, they are a useful marker as to how you are progressing. Some of these abilities give you the power to manipulate others, and many internal teachers have developed these abilities to varying degrees. At low levels, this may mean that a teacher is able to expand their energetic field so that they dominate on a very subtle, subconscious level. At higher stages, they are literally able to manipulate your thoughts and feelings through transmission directly into your mind. This gives them great power. However, if a teacher has begun to dissolve their acquired mind and bring forth the virtuous De, having power over others will seem like a ludicrous concept to them. Why on earth would you wish to dominate other people? On the other hand, if the acquired nature is still very dominant, feelings of power can easily turn a teacher into a caricature of who they used to be. Instead of the congenital nature shining forth, their acquired nature becomes stronger and stronger. Thus, these teachers may develop stronger internal energy throughout their practice while moving further and further away from their true nature. These teachers are easy to spot as they are loud and obnoxious; they tend to be emotionally unstable and to like money a lot. Many of these teachers bully their students and teach through domination.

Daoism is something of a double-edged sword. Its internal practices are powerful and, for the most part, have been well preserved; however, they lack ethical guidance and teachings on why certain practices are important. I personally have felt the alluring feel of having power over others when I first started teaching but was lucky enough to have the guidance from people I trusted to be able to step away from this and balance out my practice with exercises that cultivated my inner nature. When I first started teaching, I went on a bit of a power trip. In the end, I had to step away from teaching for several months to be in isolation and work on myself. I did not like who I was becoming. While I am still far from perfect, I think my motives are purer than they were then. As a practitioner of the internal arts, it is your responsibility to work on your nature and to keep it in constant check (especially if you teach those arts).

This kind of work is not really for those with a casual interest in the arts or for those purely interested in improving their health. This kind of work is for those who are fully committed to their practice and to the Daoist arts. This only concerns a small minority of people, for whom prolonged hours of daily training never feels like a chore. People will often claim to practise for many hours each day; however, experience has shown me that this is not really the case. Only rare individuals have the commitment to spend the necessary hours, days, months and years to go deep into the art of Daoism. This is fine though; there is no need for everybody to train in this way. It is better if most people study to the level they are able to. Life commitments often get in the way; besides, people have other interests in life that take up their time.

By way of a conclusion, I wish to discuss the necessity of sacrifice for people who get to the stage of engaging with this kind of internal work. I am speaking from personal experience, and feel it would be unfair to introduce these practices without giving the full picture of what is involved. Those wishing to try and awaken the spinal fires should be fully aware of what this entails with regards to your psyche. As each of these fires begins to awaken, it causes a great shift in your personal identity and you literally change as a person in a very short space of time. The period of change is always difficult; however, after the change has taken place, you will settle into your new way of being until the next stage of change takes place. These shifts in your personality can change the things you like, the things you place importance on and the feelings you have for those around you. As you can imagine, this can affect your relationships with other people and be extremely difficult for your loved ones. As the first fire awakens, you often find that what you are doing is wrong for you. It is common for people to walk out of their careers and sell their homes to pursue something more meaningful. This can cause problems with family and partners, as they inevitably view this kind of behaviour as self-destructive. They may even view it as slightly insane.

As each fire awakens, deeper changes take place within you, and each of these can cause problems. As I engaged with this process several years ago, I went through a very long period of rather uncomfortable changes. These changes cost me a house, a career I was going through alongside my training, a marriage and a great many other things. For a long time, it seemed as if my entire life was falling apart piece by piece. While this was difficult at the time, things have settled down now and my life is much more pleasant. I am much happier with the person I am now and glad that I shed the things in my life that were not right for me.

I am writing this because I feel it is important for people to be aware of the kind of process inherent in the internal arts. I was lucky to have no major commitments, such as children depending on me. If I had gone through these changes and destroyed a marriage with children being involved, there would have been a high chance of me negatively affecting their lives, which would not have been fair. Those practising the internal arts should take stock of what they have in their lives and, if necessary, stop before reaching these stages. You must make your art work alongside your life, unless you are prepared for the sacrifices that will result from deep internal changes.

These practices used to be kept up in the mountains, away from the masses. The ancients practised behind closed doors, keeping these practices hidden. Only those inducted into the lineages had access to the internal arts; much of this secrecy has now gone. Practices once earned through years of diligent study with a master are now available online or in chapters such as this! While this is a good thing, as it gives many people access to exercises that can improve their lives, it can also be negative. Bringing these hidden methods into the public arena incurs a certain responsibility for practitioners and teachers of the internal arts. In many ways, isolation is much easier than living in society with a family and responsibilities. For this reason, we must recognise what the risks are and weigh them up and make our practice work alongside everything else we hold dear. Only then will a lifetime study of the Daoist arts be a positive and enriching experience for everybody involved.

In conclusion, remember that any practice within the internal arts is a step-by-step process. At first, any exercise you study will seem as if it just takes place on a physical level but, with time, the exercises will begin to lead you deeper into your own being. All the Daoist arts were developed in this manner; as such, they are windows into the lives of the great teachers who came before us. To me, this makes those arts very special, and, as such, I always try to treat each exercise I have learnt as if it is special. If I treat those arts with respect and study them with the same dedication as those people who created them, then I trust they will help me develop in the correct direction.

In this chapter, I have outlined some of the risks inherent to the Daoist arts. I only wanted to make it clear how powerful and life changing they can be. If Daoist exercises are practised properly and treated with respect, they can only further people's cultivation. While dedication is important, it is also important to approach those practices with a general feeling of light-heartedness. Laugh often, do not be frustrated when you find certain things difficult and enjoy the process you are going through.

19

DAOISM AND POLITICS

Damo Mitchell

Daoism is a spiritual tradition that has had a long and often bumpy relationship with governmental politics in China. It was explained to me by some of my teachers that part of the reason Daoism had fallouts at various times in history with the other two great traditions within China (Buddhism and Confucianism) was over its political views. Buddhism has arguably had the least inclination out of the three traditions to become overly embroiled in politics. This has changed somewhat with the situation in Tibet as this has forced the Dalai Lama and his subjects into the political spotlight, but prior to this Buddhism was keen to keep its teachings apart from political institutions as much as possible. Confucianism in China was very involved in the establishment of society and politics as a whole. Hierarchical structures amongst families, communities, governments and the entire society are discussed within Confucian teachings in an effort to establish some kind of national harmony. Daoism is quite unlike Buddhism in that it was never shy of commenting on, nor getting involved in, political situations and stands in direct contrast to Confucianism, as it views all of the structures imposed by Confucius and his followers as unnatural and therefore against the way of Dao.

Many people read Daoist classical texts and view them as pure philosophical writings when in actual fact they are clear alchemical texts as well. The *Dao De Jing* itself includes a great deal of information on seated meditation methods, whilst the *Zhuangzi* (莊子) (inner chapters) also discusses health practices such as Dao Yin training. On top of this there are also countless references to the way in which a country should be run and how involved a ruler should be in the affairs of the people. Now, of course, many scholars of the *Dao De Jing* will at this stage point out that the discussion of a country is metaphorical for the practitioner's inner environment and the people discussed are the emotions that energetically exist within this environment. This is true, but Daoism works on the premise that that which occurs within the macrocosm of the outside world is directly reflected within our own personal microcosm and vice versa. In this manner Daoists do not separate teachings on our own internal being from the outer world and its political situations.

Throughout history Daoist masters were involved in political action, they advised various political rulers and they have even directly opposed emperors' decisions at various stages in time. A great many people have drawn comparisons between Daoism and anarchism, and in part this is true. If we are to bring Daoism's views on politics down to a few clear pointers we could say they are as follows.

- Governments should stay out of the lives of people as much as possible, as rules restrict freedom to grow.

- The threat of punishment and governance does not really work, as it generates rebellion and struggle, so instead aim to assist the people in attaining some kind of personal liberation.

- All people are equal, so although some kind of hierarchical system may well be required, it should be limited to what is absolutely necessary.

- Those in the lowest places should be respected and helped to find their way to Dao.

- Warfare always leads to imbalance and sadness, so it should be avoided at all costs.

- Those in charge of a people should be there only if they are benevolent people who work for the good of others; those in charge should never be the ones who seek personal gain and profit.

If you read through the *Dao De Jing* and other classical texts from the Daoist tradition you will find that these pointers come up time and time again. Unlike the Confucian teachers who sought control on every level, the Daoists wanted liberation from any outside influence that was unnecessary, as it would not help them in their search for the evolution of consciousness. The compassionate requirement of the tradition stated that they should help those around them to also live in a state of potential growth, and so restrictions put in place by overlords and such like should be spoken out against.

The reason that this is important to me as a practitioner of the Daoist arts is that I do not live in complete seclusion. Though I spend periods of time each year in isolation, I am not a full recluse. I live in a house, with a partner; I have friends and students around me a lot of the time; and I basically have to interact with the outside world fairly regularly. What this means is that I come into contact with life, people and situations that are affected greatly by politics and the decision making of those who rule our countries. In my mind, this means I cannot simply shut politics out of my life and turn a blind eye to it. This is quite different from many practitioners of meditation and similar arts that I have contact with. In many cases, when politics is mentioned, they simply reply that they do not get involved. They choose to ignore it. They are often quite surprised at just how politically opinionated I can be and how much of an interest I take in it. Many times I have caused them surprise, and some have even reminded me that 'all of life is simply an illusion' and what takes place is simply 'the Karma of those involved'. Since it is all an illusion I should 'rise above it' and get on with my practice. The 'Karma' argument always confuses me as, first, it seems like a mightily oversimplified understanding of the meaning of Karma and, second, it seems very unjust to take this view and then apply it to those who are suffering on a daily basis around you because of difficulties within our society. 'I am sorry you are starving hungry and about to lose your home – it must be your Karma!' I am not sure I would be too prepared to tell anybody that.

Now, if I am perfectly honest, political shifts within my own government do not affect me a great deal. Whilst certainly not rich, I am not poor either. I have no fear of my employment situation being changed, as I work for myself and teach the internal arts as a professional teacher. In short, I guess I would generally be placed into what we know as the 'middle class' with regards to my position within society. This means that if I wished to I could have the luxury of taking this same stance of completely ignoring politics and simply focusing upon my own life and training. This has not always been the case though, and I have certainly experienced the difficulties of life from the position of somebody living at the bottom of the socio-economic ladder.

The problem with simply ignoring such difficulties because I am now 'fine' is that my life situation is not the same as those around me. I have friends and other people within my life who are not in the same socio-economic situation, and so shifting politics do have a direct and major effect upon them. If benefits are reduced or wages are cut by the government then this can have a major impact upon their existence. Many people are living in constant fear that they are going to lose their home to ever-tightening financial laws that are making the cost of living almost impossible to attain. On top of this the homeless situation is ever-increasing and people on the 'bottom' rungs of our societal and financial ladder are constantly suffering. Is this their Karma? Maybe, maybe not. I don't have the answer to this, as I don't believe that anybody who has not yet reached an enlightened state of being could ever really be in a position of understanding such high-minded concepts.

Let us look at another factor within the state of human existence. This is the issue of attaining some kind of personal liberation. Now, not all people are aiming for the same thing. Some are looking for happiness, others for some kind of meaning in their life and then, of course, there are the 'full on' practitioners aiming to alchemically transform themselves into spiritual immortals! Whatever the goal, high minded or fairly mundane, not many people have the express aim in life of suffering as much as they can, and so I would guess that most want at least to be content in some way or another. Now, as a follower of Daoism, I have been informed that the macrocosm of the outside world and the microcosm of my inner being are inextricably linked. I am also of the opinion that it would be great if everybody in the world was able to get to a stage whereby they could also engage in some kind of personal transformative arts. Meditation for all people would be great but unrealistic – I would simply settle for the *option* of meditation for all.

A commonly referred to psychological model is Maslow's hierarchy of needs. This model is shown in Figure 19.1. It shows the order that a person's needs should be met if they are to attain what Maslow called a state of self-actualisation.

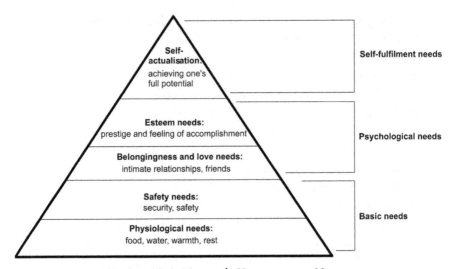

FIGURE 19.1: MASLOW'S HIERARCHY OF NEEDS

At the bottom of the pyramid are physiological needs, which in this case mean basic requirements such as adequate food, shelter and so on. If a person does not have these basic needs met then they are not able to focus upon anything apart from these immediate issues. Above this is the need for safety, which also includes security within any societal system. There must be an adequate level of support and financial security for people in their life to prevent the constant stress of entering into a state of poverty. Next on the list is the requirement for feeling loved or like you 'belong'. Politically I see this as the importance of an acceptant and non-judgemental society where all are welcome, no matter their gender, social class, nationality, asylum status or sexual orientation. Those who do not have a feeling of belonging are likely to be 'distracted' psychologically by this issue, which will hold them back from 'moving up the pyramid'. Self-esteem is next on the list. This can seem like a strange step on the way towards self-actualisation through the Daoist arts, as ultimately a person is aiming to dissolve a 'sense of self'. Whilst this is true, I pose the question: can a person realistically dissolve their acquired self unless that sense of self is in a position of strength with regards to self-esteem? From what I have seen, when there is a very low self-esteem and a person engages with meditative training, some students are okay whilst many others actually find that the practice damages their level of self-worth even more. This is a great challenge for teachers of these arts – how do we build up a person's self-confidence and self-esteem whilst at the same time trying to help a person see through the illusion of self? I put it to you that there is no easy answer to this issue and that those who think there is a simple resolution may well be ignoring the various complexities of the human condition.

The model shows us that only when these basic conditions have been met may a person attain some kind of self-actualisation, which in the case of the Daoist arts refers to engaging in an effective practice that will help a person to attain conscious evolution or, at least, some kind of inner peace. Of course this is just a model, and so many people will engage with Daoism prior to meeting all of these needs, but in the end I believe that those who are at least in a position to have these needs met are more likely to gain stronger results from the practice.

Why is this relevant to politics with regards to Daoism? The reason it is important is that it is the nation's politics that have the greatest and most immediate effect upon the lower-tier needs of a person's life. For this reason I stand with whatever political party/candidate seems to be most in support of the people at the absolute bottom of our society with regards to their needs and social standing. Those that speak out for social inclusion and assistance for those struggling are the ones that most align themselves with the philosophy of the Dao. This is not for myself, as I don't really have issues within the 'lower tier' of the pyramid. Like the other meditation practitioners I mentioned above, my life is actually quite secure and so I can engage happily with my practice. Instead it is for the people in the world around me. It is for those living within the macrocosm of which I am a part. To ignore the needs of those around you is both selfish in my opinion as well as somewhat ignorant of the interconnected nature of all. It often disheartens me just how many political leaders seem to harp on at great length about how their policies will help the 'middle classes' of the country. In this manner they garner a great deal of support from those who are already doing fairly well in life whilst those at the bottom are, at best, ignored and sadly often demonised within the media. As a society it is those in immediate risk who should be helped, even if it is at the slight cost of those who are more secure. According to the *Dao De Jing* (Verse 8) 'Dao flows to the lowest places', and so should human compassion.

On another level, I am never in favour of any laws that seek to impose rules, increase surveillance or restrict the freedoms of people.

As the ancient Daoists made clear, freedom is more likely to occur when there is less in the way of governance. Systems and such like are against the way of Dao. As a follower of the Daoist path, freedom is of paramount importance to me. Freedom comes from living in a society where minimal involvement comes from those in charge for those who don't require any assistance. Freedom does not come at the removal of rights nor from bombs dropped by Western imperialist powers. It comes from a system where all people within a society are valued and assisted with whatever needs they may have to reach a state of non-physical suffering; only then can the search for non-psychological suffering begin. In short, is politics the biggest driving force within my personal life? No, my practice is. But I would never be so foolish as to think that politics play no part in my life or the lives of those around me. Change in people needs to come from inside, sure, but it also needs to happen for many people on a physical, practical level too. Even if physical life is simply an illusion, it is a pretty darn uncomfortable one for many...

20

MARTIAL ARTS – REALM OF THE INSECURE
Damo Mitchell

Let us always be brutally honest with ourselves as to why we started training in the martial arts in the first place. I have spent my life around various forms of martial arts classes and practitioners. When I was younger it was within the Japanese external systems, and as I grew older it was within the Chinese systems. This means that over the years I have grown to know many people who started training in different forms of Gong Fu (功夫). Some of those people are still training, whilst the vast majority have since stopped and moved on to other things. One thing that always fascinated me is the common thread that pulled all of those people into martial training, which is both arduous and longwinded. Why would somebody wish to dedicate so much time to painstakingly analysing every little facet of their body movement through the medium of combat? Now, with the exception of those who got into something like Taijiquan for health reasons, I see that the vast majority began training because they were deeply insecure.

This insecurity may have come about for various reasons. In many cases a person was bullied or physically threatened in some way, which is one of the most difficult things for the human psyche to ever come to terms with. In some cases people were insecure because they were physically frail and martial arts seemed like a good way to become strong. I have met some who were insecure because of the way in which they had been brought up by their parents, and even those who felt insecure because they naturally lacked grace and poise. I feel that if the majority of us looked inside we would see that our training also came from a sense of deep insecurity, which was or is leaving a gaping hole in our inner being.

If I look at myself as an example I can understand this situation very well. I began training at age four because I was sent to the classes by my parents. At this age I was blissfully unaware of the stresses of life and so no major insecurities had developed. Consequently, I was not much interested in the arts and so I treated them as a casual hobby, somewhere I went in the evenings to play and throw my arms and legs in the air. This all changed as I got older and began to realise that other people possibly posed a threat. I have always been slight in stature, and as a child and young teen it made me a target for bullying. Here was the seed of insecurity that left its mark and drove me into a serious study of Karate-Do and then the Chinese systems. This insecurity has carried me through years of continuous training, and though I am close to dealing with my inner turmoil it is always a long journey – the mind is always reluctant to let go of the deepest injuries.

The problem with these kinds of psychological aspects is that they tend to dictate each and every thing that we do. Our inner state becomes the standpoint from which we experience the outside world. It causes us to emotionally distort the way in which we act as our damaged psyche seeks to defend itself from further hurt. The spiritual traditions of the East have long understood this and so developed various systems of self-cultivation, which would enable a person to deal with their own being and so elevate themselves to a higher state. Martial arts was one such tool, or at least it has the potential to be so if used correctly.

There is an inherent difficulty within the martial arts world and that is that the most insecure are the people who stay within the arts the longest. They are the ones whose inner nature sees the potential for change, even if they don't consciously understand what this crazy drive is that borders on obsession. This means that, almost inevitably, they become the teachers of the arts – those with the most experience and the most years of dedicated effort put into the arts. By the very nature of what it means to be a teacher, students will come to you and then look to you for guidance. On the surface they may be looking to you for martial technique, but subconsciously they are also looking for something else – a way to deal with that same insecurity that most likely led their newfound teacher into the arts in the first place. This is a responsibility that all teachers need to recognise and take on board.

It was for these reasons that, classically, schools of martial arts, especially internal practices, would teach ethics alongside their arts. The view was basically that a person could be measured by their actions and the state of their Heart-Mind, not by the strength of their punch. Sadly, over the years this message was lost and, in my opinion, the ethics of martial arts are all but dead. Gong Fu has reached an all-time low of morality, etiquette and self-cultivation. Take a journey onto any martial arts forum and see the countless pages of arguments to see how true this is.

As practitioners (and certainly as teachers) we need to remember that it was a deep-rooted insecurity that initially led us to these practices and that almost everybody in this community is coming from the same place. At this point maybe your brain is going, 'Rubbish, I am not insecure – what is he talking about?' If this is the case I would suggest that maybe you are one of the lucky few who are perfectly balanced or perhaps you need to look a little deeper inside and be a bit more honest with yourself.

Why this is important is because if you constantly trash others and attack them either physically or verbally you are essentially damaging the other person's inner nature. Their insecurity is likely to become deeper no matter how hard they try to shake off what has been said or done. Each step towards weakening that person's inner nature is taking away from their development. Two people will enter into a conflict because one or both is trying to come to terms with their own insecurity. In order to validate their own stance and thus defend their fragile ego, they will argue until one is the perceived victor and one the loser. The 'winner' has confirmed the distorted viewpoint of his own nature in his own mind, whilst the 'loser' has been damaged even more deeply. This is certainly not an effective method of inner growth for either party. In modern times this is made even worse by the internet and martial arts forums. Here, insecure people can shout at others and try to validate their position whilst gathering around them other insecure people to prop up their fragile egos. A gathering of wounded egos attacking each other through typed words should be avoided at all costs lest the inner-growth aspect of martial arts be lost forever.

This is why I never support martial arts competitions. In each case there must always be a 'winner' and a 'loser'. If, in a perfect world, competitions or challenges were between two people who mutually accepted that they were there to better their arts and themselves then competition could be a good thing. After a couple of years of taking part in martial arts tournaments I realised that this was sadly not the case. With each win my ego validated my own standpoint whether I was in the right or the wrong, and with each loss my sense of insecurity was etched more deeply into my being. With each competition I see, I witness the same process going on whether the participants are aware of this or not. Martial arts should abhor this kind of practice. In life you should never compete, but, at the same time, if you must fight you should not lose. Not losing and being competitive are not the same thing, and I believe more martial artists should spend time contemplating the differences between these two. This is the heart of the study that we undertake.

I don't write this as a rant or an attack but as a thought process that I have been through lately after reading a few martial arts forums and seeing the processes taking place there. A martial arts forum is not somewhere you will ever see me contributing in any great length simply because I find the dynamics of what is taking place in these communities counter-productive to what I am seeking – inner development through the medium of martial arts study. I would urge sincere practitioners of a like mind to question themselves and their motives before getting involved in such places, as the ethical side of study needs to come back lest martial arts become a pale shadow of what they once were. Let us work together to further ourselves and our arts, not fight over things that really bear no importance to the nature of our inner development. A sense of insecurity can become the greatest fuel for a lifetime journey of self-cultivation and development or it can, sadly, lead us onto a path of egoistic distortion that helps nobody. That choice is ultimately ours alone.

21

THE PINEAL GLAND AND DAOISM

Damo Mitchell

It is interesting to note that many different cultures around the world and throughout history have placed great importance upon the pineal gland with regards to their spiritual practice. Almost without exception, the pineal gland has appeared within the teachings of different ancient groups who assigned the cultivation of spiritual awakening to this pea-sized gland that sits deep within the brain.

In alchemical language the pineal gland is known as the Ni Wan (泥丸), that is often translated as being the 'mud pill palace'. It is the physical manifestation, the Jing, of the upper Dan Tien, which is a rotating sphere of information that serves to govern our mental faculties, movements of consciousness and level of connection to the divine. So is the pineal gland the upper Dan Tien? The answer to this is both yes and no. The upper Dan Tien manifests energetically as a sphere of Qi within the skull and physically as the pineal gland within the Ni Wan area of the head. The physical and energetic anatomy of the pineal gland is shown in Figure 21.1. Included is the brain, the pineal gland and the upper Dan Tien.

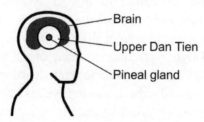

FIGURE 21.1: THE PINEAL GLAND AND UPPER DAN TIEN

The pineal gland has been discovered to react to light – photon energy – by biological scientists. This often causes confusion, as the pineal gland essentially sits within complete darkness inside the head so often it is known as the 'appendix' of the brain: a supposedly useless organ that serves little purpose. Interestingly, other studies have shown that the pineal gland secretes serotonin, which is directly involved in governing our happiness levels and preventing us from sinking into depression. The light that the pineal gland reacts to within Daoist alchemical thought is the Shen energy rising up through the Chong Mai into the area of the upper Dan Tien. As the vibratory frequency of the Shen hits the pineal gland it generates a reaction that gives the appearance of a white light appearing within the mind's eye. This light, with practice, can begin to expand itself over the head of a sincere practitioner, leading to the formation of a halo of white energy that can be perceived by those around who have awakened the spiritual eye, the collateral branch of the energy body that runs from the pineal gland to the Yin Tang area of the head, as shown in Figure 21.2. This is the equivalent of what is more commonly known as the 'third eye' or 'spiritual eye' within esoteric traditions.

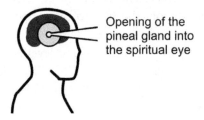

Opening of the pineal gland into the spiritual eye

FIGURE 21.2: THE SPIRITUAL EYE

The pineal gland is 'awakened' by this internal light. This leads to perception beyond the realms of physical vision. Psychic vision, abilities and phenomena can be attained once the pineal gland receives the light it requires from deep within the consciousness of the accomplished Daoist practitioner. Many of the intermediary-level abilities recorded as being available to internal arts practitioners are a result of the pineal gland – the 'all-seeing eye', as it was known within many gnostic schools – awakening and giving a glimpse of the world beyond the realm of Jing – physicality.

Beyond the pineal gland and this realm of light – Shen – lies the realm of emptiness, the gateway to Dao. It is the role of the upper

Dan Tien to convert the higher-perception frequencies of the pineal gland's by-products into a direct connection to the divine. This is now entering the higher stages of alchemical practices. Only the most ardent meditation devotees will enter this door and find the opening of the doorway to Dao.

It is fascinating to me how the pineal gland has been represented within ancient cultures. In many cases it was represented with a pine cone, as can be seen in many examples of ancient architecture, religious artefacts and even within the Vatican. I had the opportunity to visit the Vatican recently, and pineal 'cones' were frequently ornamentation. It has long been knowledge within the religious traditions of both the East and the West that the pineal gland is an important factor in any spiritual seeker's connection with the divine, but sadly this information has been largely lost.

The pineal gland then became changed into the pyramid image that we see as an important image within the majority of mystery schools and ancient orders. The pyramid image with the all-seeing eye, which appears on American money and within many symbols and logos, represents the pineal gland, the activation of the 'spiritual eye' through Shen information. It is even possible to see the white light of the pyramid surrounding meditation practitioners who are able to utilise the full lotus position in their practice. This light is directed from the upturned feet of the lotus position towards the third eye area of the head as the pineal gland begins to activate. It is easy to see how the pyramid became linked to spiritual elevation once you have witnessed the Shen triangle appear around a practitioner during internal alchemy. From these logos it is clear to see that the formation of countries and governments around the world was originally down to those with great knowledge of the internal workings of human consciousness. For many, the symbol of the all-seeing eye, as it appears in Figure 21.3, has become something of a sinister image – the mark of a growing Orwellian state. Whatever the truth now, it was originally a sign of great spiritual significance.

Problems with the pineal gland can arise if it becomes calcified to any great degree. Calcification encases the pineal gland in a hard shell much like the enamel layer surrounding our teeth. This prevents the pineal gland from receiving any spiritual light. This essentially plunges our higher consciousness into darkness and prevents us from attaining any kind of spiritual awakening. Calcification of the pineal gland can lead to depression, fatigue, muscle pain and wastage on a physical level. Many researchers are now even linking the pineal gland's calcification to numerous chronic medical conditions, though this is not widely accepted within the mainstream medical community. On top of this, it prevents meditation practitioners from moving beyond the realm of physical perception in their practice. In my opinion, it is of the utmost importance for any internal arts practitioner serious about alchemical advancement to stop consuming anything that can contribute to calcification of the pineal gland. Steps should then be taken to reverse any damage that has already been done. Thankfully, the calcification can indeed be reversed.

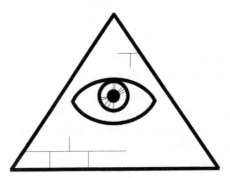

FIGURE 21.3: THE ALL-SEEING EYE

The biggest offender in calcification of the pineal gland is Fluoride. This is the toxic substance that is put into many countries' drinking water. In the past it was considered crazy to even discuss such things, and those against Fluoridation of water were quickly labelled as 'crackpot conspiracy theorists'. Thankfully, there is more of an open-minded approach being taken to questioning of this sort these days and some countries in Europe have even managed to de-fluoridate their water due to research that shows how dangerous a chemical it can be. It was always said to help prevent tooth decay, but emerging evidence shows that this is not actually the case; some have even managed to show that it does the opposite! Fluoride is also in our toothpaste, but luckily it is easy enough to buy Fluoride-free toothpaste over the internet or in many health stores. Also, be aware that many bottled drinking water companies now put Fluoride into the water as well. In the UK we are lucky enough to not have Fluoride in the majority of our towns' water supplies, but the water companies still pump Fluoride unannounced into the water to purify it if there have been reports of any contaminations to the water. Those who really want to save their pineal gland should seriously consider drinking only Fluoride-free water and avoiding Fluoride-laden toothpaste. I have even suggested this to several people who suffer with clinical depression and their depression has gone away within a couple of weeks. It is my opinion that many cases of depression are actually linked to calcification of the pineal gland due to Fluoride poisoning. If you are reading this and you suffer from depression, try switching your toothpaste and monitoring your water to ensure that it is pure; see what happens.

Processed foods and (research is suggesting) GMO foods also attack the pineal gland, as well as numerous other aspects of our mind and body. These should be cut out of the diet in order to protect the pineal gland's functioning.

Organic food helps to heal the pineal gland. Especially important are organic green leafy vegetables that have a strong de-calcifying effect upon the body in general. Spirulina is very useful, along with Goji berries. Both are great foods for meditation practitioners. I have also read recently that fermented cod-liver oil is also great for helping the pineal gland, but I have not had the chance to try this yet. Also remember to drink plenty of pure water in order to detoxify the system and cleanse the blood.

Those who practise the Heavenly Streams exercises in my books can also help the pineal gland to de-calcify by focusing upon the GV17 point 'Nao Hu' (腦戶) or the GV24 point 'Shen Ting' (神庭) and activating them in the same way as described for other points in the *Heavenly Streams: Meridian Theory in Nei Gong* book. Practise with these points for around five minutes a day and you should help your poor pineal gland greatly! These points are shown in Figure 21.4.

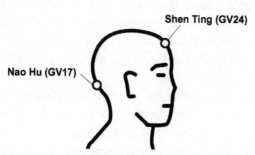

FIGURE 21.4: NAO HU AND SHEN TING

22

SUNG AND ENERGETIC RELAXATION

Damo Mitchell

Anybody beginning their study of Qi Gong will no doubt have been told to either 'relax', 'let go' or, in Chinese, 'Sung/Song' (松). Though seemingly an easy instruction, it is in fact one of the most difficult aspects of the internal arts. Rather than simply being an instruction that may be carried out immediately, it is a continual process of releasing and then reconnecting, which becomes a gradual and constant part of any Qi Gong practitioner's daily regime.

Through teaching the process of Sung within Qi Gong classes it has struck me time and again just how difficult it is for many people to go 'Sung', especially those new to the internal arts, and also how much confusion there is over the process of 'letting go'.

Relaxing the body has to take place on the same three key levels as the rest of Daoist training. Relaxation must first appear within the physical body; from here it is the energetic body that then needs to release its tensions/blockages. These two then form a continuous loop of releasing more tension in order to allow the other to release deeper, and in this way the cycle of going Sung builds deeper and deeper into the core of your being. These two then, in turn, rely on relaxation of the mind, which can be the most difficult for many people, as this requires deep levels of inner searching and letting go of the mind's attachments, projections and motivations. This cycle of Sung is shown in Figure 22.1.

Sung must take place for there to be effective energetic flow within the body even if we ignore all of the obvious physical benefits to relaxing the mind and body. Without an adequate level of Sung being reached it is highly unlikely that any real levels of personal transformation can be managed, as the information highway of the meridian system will be stuck or flow with a 'roughness' that is not conducive to gaining results in your practice.

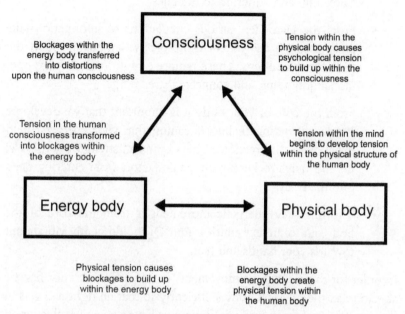

FIGURE 22.1: THE CYCLE OF SUNG

If we had to summarise the key energetic flows that are aimed for within the body they would be as follows.

- The Qi within the torso needs to sink down towards the lower abdomen so that the natural focal point within your body is the lower abdominal region.

- Within this downward flow there needs to be a strong upwards flow through the central channel of the body and up the governing meridian, which runs through the centre of your back.

- The downward flow within your torso then needs to extend down towards the ground where it meets the opposite flow of Qi rising from the planet up through Yong Quan (涌泉) towards the lower Dan Tien.

- As the Qi from the upper part of your torso reaches the lower abdomen some of it flows towards your back where it spreads via the shape of your Trapezius to give you an energetic movement that corresponds to the classical principle of 'spreading and adhering to the back'.

- From the Dan Tien various circulations of information take place through the microcosmic orbits that run through the torso, arms and legs. These require a high level of relaxation, fascial unbinding and connected stretching.

- From the core of your body it is important that we develop a gentle expanding feeling, meaning that your energetic field expands in all directions. This expansion strengthens the Wei Qi and helps to keep pathogenic factors from entering deep into the body.

- The final key energetic movement is from the core of the body out to the extremities. Your Qi should gently vibrate out towards your hands and feet.

In order for these energetic movements to take place we must first be able to relax the physical body sufficiently so that no tightness gets in the way. Physical tension or misalignments have a negative effect upon our energetic flow that curiously has both a vibratory and a slightly fluid nature to it.

Relaxing the physical body correctly involves understanding the principle of letting go with the muscles whilst at the same time connecting the soft tissues together into a single unit.

The soft tissues of the body can connect together into one single unit that takes the form of a kind of 'biological wetsuit', providing we understand how to utilise a correct bodily posture in our practice. The Qi Gong structure is designed to allow this 'wetsuit' to spread out and link into a single unit, meaning that any movement within a part of the body has a direct effect upon every other part of the body. Correct connection means that if we carry out a simple motion, such as extending a finger, we will feel this movement carried across the rest of the body. This is obviously an important attainment for anybody studying the internal martial arts of Taijiquan, Xingyiquan or Baguazhang, as well as Qi Gong. Not only this, but the connectivity goes deep inside of the body as well. Our connective tissues run not only on the surface but also deep inside the body right through to the fascia surrounding each of our organs and down to the surface of our bones. A high level of connection means that any movement with our physical body will also result in gentle pulls and motions deep within our core. This has profound ramifications upon the level of our physical health, as any motion we make will then begin to purge the internal organs of stagnant fluids and energetic pathogens that may have collected around them. If we wish to summarise the importance of Sung for connection we can simply state that tension generates contraction and contraction generates disconnection.

In order to connect this 'wetsuit' together into a whole, we must learn how to let the major muscle groups of the body go soft and 'hang' from the bones. As this happens, the level of habitual contraction held within our body will release, and this will in turn create more potential for expansion. As we release the tension we can begin to gently pull out the soft tissues using our fingers and toes as the extremes of these stretches. This stretch needs to be long, even and spread across the whole body. Do not overstretch to the point where tension is created though, as this will begin to work against the Sung process. Remember that 'what you train is what you become', so continued overstretching to the point of tension will actually disconnect your body and make you more tense in both body and mind. This is a common issue that I see within the internal arts; people are often either too slack, which creates stagnation, or too taut, which produces tension and blockages.

The result of this process is that as you gradually release more, you will find that you begin to 'disconnect'. The soft tissues of your outer being will begin to become slack unless you increase the level of stretch across the body. You are aiming to get to the stage whereby your outer surface, becomes 'like the skin of a drum'. This is an important analogy, as the skin of a drum enables vibrations to pass along its surface, and this is what we want to happen within our own body. The 'drum skin' of our 'biological wetsuit' is required to be in such a state of connection that it enables the vibratory information of our Qi to pass through it. This is the key method of bringing our internal energy from our core and expressing it within the external world – whether this be for martial, therapeutic or spiritual reasons.

As the body gradually releases more tension, we can begin to open up the most difficult line within our body that runs from our hips or Kua (胯) region down to the ground and the base of our feet, as shown in Figure 22.2.

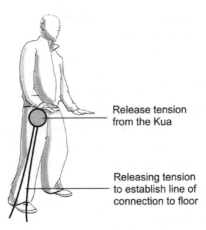

Release tension
from the Kua

Releasing tension
to establish line of
connection to floor

FIGURE 22.2: THE KUA AND FEET LINE OF CONNECTION

By opening this line we develop root and enable energetic flow up from the ground into our body. Particular focus should be applied to this region of the body when practising Sung, as it is here that dictates whether or not we will connect effectively with the planet. About 80 per cent of people who I teach actually 'hold on' with their buttocks without realising during any standing Qi Gong work, and this is obviously a major block to the process of Sung within the lower body.

If you manage to connect successfully with this Sung process you will then discover that the gradual extension of the soft tissues begins to transmit mechanical information into the core of the body; now your adjustments will begin to pull and stretch open the inside of the body automatically, giving you the feeling that small movements are taking place inside of your skeletal structure. What is happening is that your 'biological wetsuit' is now starting to pull the bones into a more efficient alignment through micro-adjustments that it would be impossible for you to make correctly if you tried using your conscious mind. It is more effective to allow the process of Sung to make these adjustments for you as you release and reconnect to ever-more efficient levels.

At this stage it is possible to start integrating practices such as Sung Breathing; this practice can be read about in my book on Daoist Nei Gong (*Daoist Nei Gong: The Philosophical Art of Change*). This will then help the body to remember this state through adjusting the plasticity of the soft tissues into a more effective structure. Through conscious connection of your breathing to your body's energetic movements it is possible to create a kind of 'liquid wave' of Qi that moves through the soft tissues and vibrates out along the 'wetsuit' you have created. It is at this stage that the 'drum skin' principle becomes particularly important. The 'drum skin' of the soft tissues can be thought of as a kind of 'conductor' for the movement of Qi.

The alignment that your body has been put in by this process then begins to adjust your energetic flow to match the key movement principles outlined in the bullet points above. As this happens it is wise to simply allow your mind to gently attach to the movements and observe what is taking place. Through giving your energy body a little attention you will enable it to work more efficiently, and so the whole process of Sung will take place on a stronger level within the energetic body. You may observe this for some time, but eventually you will reach the stage where it feels as if this energetic growth can go no further. This is the point where you must re-enter the physical Sung process and work towards making your connection and micro-adjustments even more efficient. When you think you can Sung no more – Sung some more.

Throughout all of this work it is likely that your body will begin to shed some of its imbalances. The physical body can begin to unbind any tensions stored within the physical tissues, resulting in feelings of deep bruises; do not worry about this – these are just blockages opening up and passing. They will not last long. Note though that these deep bruises are just that – bruised feelings, not sharp pains. If you get sharp pains then it is likely that you have an incorrect alignment somewhere within your structure that needs resolving before you cause any further injury. Be particularly aware of these misalignments around the region of your knees and spine, as when damaged they can take a long time to repair.

As the energy body releases stagnation it is likely that you will begin to shake or vibrate, sometimes quite violently. If this happens do not worry – it is quite normal; simply release more against it and allow more space for the energy to come out through. When this has been achieved you will find that the shake becomes a more steady and smooth wave that does not cause such violent reactions for your body. These releases are often accompanied by emotional release, which can result in random laughing fits or tears; again, do not worry – simply allow them to pass, as they are a sign of your body making adjustments to itself through your Sung process.

This has been an introduction to the early stages of Sung; there is a great deal more to the process, but I hope these pointers will help some people to begin exploring this often-overlooked aspect of the internal arts. From here there is the Sung process of the mind, which is the gateway to achieving varying states of stillness, but that is a long topic. It is also something I do not recommend undertaking without the guidance of a trusted teacher, as the process can sometimes be difficult for people, both technically and emotionally.

Never be satisfied with the amount of Sung you have achieved – relax, connect more, relax more, connect more; this is the way to attaining Sung. It is not a quick or easy process, but rather something that becomes a lifelong study in its own right.

23

FOOD ENERGETICS
Damo Mitchell

When teaching internal arts there is one particular question that arises time and time again. This is the question of: 'What should a person eat in order to be healthy and assist in their practice?'

The subject of food and healthy eating is a very large one. There are countless books written on different diets, the correct way to balance your nutritional intake and, of course, how to make sure you don't gain excess weight. If you have ever taken the time to look at the nutrition section of any bookshop you will have seen that there are countless views that generally seem to contradict each other. Each week a new diet comes out based on the latest research – a situation that does not make the subject of healthy eating any easier to tackle.

Chinese medicine also has very clear teachings on how a person should eat in order to stay healthy; these teachings are a part of the wider subject of Yang Sheng Fa or 'life-nourishing methods'. If we look at what 'life-nourishing methods' means, it is simply 'healthy living'. The medical viewpoint of the ancient Chinese was greatly influenced by the Daoist tradition and in particular the energetic/Tantric theories of the alchemical practitioners. Almost identical theories underpin Chinese herbal medicine and, as such, the idea is that 'food is fuel or medicine'. For myself, that is the first idea that I try to teach my students. Whilst there is absolutely nothing wrong with enjoying the taste of your food, do not make this the most important factor when deciding what you will eat. Taste is simply one of our senses and, essentially, we should not be allowing the temporary pleasure of our senses to dictate what we do. Too many people decide their diet by what they 'like to eat', and consequently we have a generation of people addicted to sugary and processed foods. On top of this we have created countless chemical formulas that aim to make our flavours stronger and stronger until often you cannot even remember what a

163

particular item of food was supposed to taste like in the first place! The simple rule is that 'what you put in you get out'. The body runs on the food we eat, and if we really wish to be healthy and get the most out of our internal practices we must eat in a healthy and balanced manner.

With particular regards to practitioners of the internal arts there is also another aspect of healthy eating we should keep in mind. When a person begins to practise an art such as Qi Gong, Nei Gong, meditation or Yoga they are essentially strengthening the relationship that exists between body and mind. Through repeatedly bringing our awareness into either our body or the processes taking place within it, we are increasing the efficiency of our own personal interface. According to Daoist thought, the medium through which this interface is experienced is our Qi. The bond between mind and physicality grows through suffusion of Qi through more of our being as well as a releasing of our awareness into this particular energetic state. This becomes something of a double-edged sword with regards to our health. This is because when we eat food that has a direct effect upon the quality of our energy, it generates a far more potent reaction within our mind and body than if we were not internal practitioners. I have seen people come into the internal arts who have never bothered regulating their diet. They have been living on burgers, pizzas, processed foods and drinking a lot of alcohol on the weekends. Despite their diet they have been fairly robust; sure, they may have been carrying a few extra pounds, but in general they were continuing with their lives, sustaining themselves in this way. As soon as they start to work with the internal arts they suddenly experience a massive drop in their health. They become sick, they age quickly and they gain a lot of weight. This is extremely common, though sometimes the connection between the practice and the change in the person's health is not noticed. In some cases the opposite is true: the changes are noticed and the practitioner blames the internal system for the problem; they claim that the practice is dangerous and has made them sick. In actual fact, this is half true and half false. The system of practice has indeed been involved in the drop in their health but only because of the increased power of the food to affect them on a deep level. As these changes take place within the energetic flow, there are direct manifestations within the physical body as well as the mind, and thus the person becomes weaker. This is something that all internal practitioners should be aware of. The other side of this issue is that, of course, if a person eats healthily then the increased effects of the healthy diet becomes amplified as well. An organic, energetically rich diet, free from processed food and chemicals, will supercharge their practice as the quality of Qi generates positive changes throughout the mind/body system.

It is for these reasons that all sincere internal practitioners should look at their diet and think carefully about what they are going to eat.

Another factor to be aware of is that life is made up of conceptual models. This is sometimes a strange concept for people to get their minds around when they begin training, but to me it is an absolute. I have seen how a person's conceptual model forms their reality, time and time again. What I mean by this is that we all have theories and beliefs that shape how we see the world. In the majority of cases I would guess that readers of this book were initially brought up to see the world from a scientific viewpoint. Possibly this scientific viewpoint was also affected to a certain degree by cultural and maybe even religious beliefs. What this means is that, primarily, a person's worldview was based in the physical and the tangible, as this is where most modern education is based. When we apply this to food we have rules such as balancing of proteins, carbohydrates, vitamins and minerals. This is the basic level of study for anybody who looks at nutrition according to our modern understanding of food. Of course, this works. If a person learns how to regulate their diet according to these principles then they can understand how to get the most out of their body and thus regulate their health. This is because they are controlling their reality according to the conceptual model they see life through. This all changes, however, when people begin to study the internal arts. It is an interesting phenomenon to see that once a student begins to contact their energy body and study the nature of it, they shift into an entirely different conceptual model. As their level of contact and understanding grows they generally find that they need to make changes to their lifestyle in order to match the new paradigm their consciousness is working to. Whereas their previous diet based upon Western nutritional theory worked for them, they now find that they are not being sustained in the same way. Instead they generally feel that they need to shift away from this way of working towards a diet that is more suitable to their energetic system. I feel that I need to point this out in this chapter, as I have seen many students fall into the trap of not understanding how much their conceptual model of life governs every aspect of their being. Whilst Western nutrition is still important, the internal arts practitioner generally finds benefit from understanding the nature of food energetics according to ancient Chinese teachings.

The Chinese energetic view of food is that all food can be categorised into five main types. These are Hot foods, Warm foods, Neutral foods, Cool foods and Cold foods. Each of these categories primarily concerns the way in which the food causes energy to move within the body. The movement of Qi through our internal environment causes changes to the information moving through our system, and so this in turn produces various effects within us. These changes govern the balance of Yin and Yang, which is the foundation of all aspects of health according to Daoism. Let us look at each of the five energetic food categories individually.

ENERGETIC FOOD CATEGORIES

Hot Foods

Hot foods are also sometimes known as Fire foods. These are foods that contain the energy of extreme expansion and rising. When we eat these foods the resulting energy of the food causes our Qi to rise upwards within the body and expand outwards, as shown in Figure 23.1. This is not generally considered a healthy movement of Qi for the majority of people.

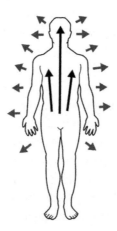

FIGURE 23.1: THE MOVEMENT OF HOT FOOD ENERGY

As the Qi rises up in the body it causes a shift towards a Yang state. This, if continued for too long or too often, damages the foundation of Yin, leading to the potential for many imbalances. Anything that causes Qi to rise and expand will raise the body's temperature, burn up fluids and generally excite the mind. The key organs of the body to become affected are the Liver and the Heart, which always react to these kinds of energetic shifts. In order to deal with this kind of energy it is also common for the Kidneys to try to harmonise your system, which they do by governing the Heart's Fire. This puts pressure on the Kidneys' Qi, which can become drained if the body is subject to these kinds of energetic effects for too long.

Hot foods are a large category within our modern diet. This is because as well as the various foods that naturally fall into this category, we also have all foods that are high in sugar and chemicals and those foods that are highly processed. Any quick look around a supermarket will show you just how much Hot food is on offer to us in modern society. After a certain stage has been reached in internal work it is quite clear to feel the negative effects these foods are having upon the body.

As a general rule, Hot foods should be consumed rarely, and in the case of those people who are already Yin deficient should be avoided altogether. They are also negative foods to eat during the summer or on particularly warm days, as this will cause too much Yang to arise. At the end of this chapter are some example lists of foods that fall into each of the five energetic categories.

Warm Foods

Warm foods obviously have some of the same energetic properties as Hot foods but not to such extreme levels. Warm foods also generate rising and expanding energetic movements when we consume them but they do not cause imbalance within the body, nor do they drain the Kidneys in any way. Expansion is required within the energy body in order to generate change. These changes include all energetic functional activities of the organs, tissues and even the cells of the body. This warmth is the catalyst for all life, and so consequently within ancient Chinese thought this was a very positive category of food. It is for this reason that Chinese medicine practitioners will often advise a person to try and avoid eating too many cold salads. Though they are often viewed as healthy food within Western thought, salads are not considered to have the necessary energetic components to generate the catalyst of warm, expanding energy within us. Figure 23.2 shows the energetic movement of Warm foods when we consume them.

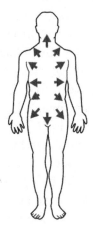

FIGURE 23.2: THE MOVEMENT OF WARM FOOD ENERGY

Seasonally, winter was considered to be a difficult time for the body to generate the energy it requires to sustain efficient functioning. The body simply does not have any help from the environmental Qi, which is naturally contracting during this time period. For this reason it was advised that the vast majority of a person's food should come from the Warm category and all Cool and Cold foods be avoided as much as possible.

Neutral Foods

Neutral foods cause energy to shift within the body but not to such a dramatic rate as any of the other four categories. These foods cause Qi to circulate around the body but do not cause expansion within the system. Figure 23.3 shows the movement of Qi caused by neutral foods.

These are healthy energetic foods to consume, as they have no leaning towards either Yin or Yang, but if a person were only to consume neutral foods then there would be a lack of drive in the system due to a lack of added expansion. Generally, these foods are exempt from any seasonal rules and as such can be consumed all year round.

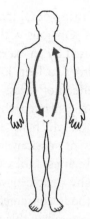

FIGURE 23.3: THE MOVEMENT OF NEUTRAL FOOD ENERGY

Cool Foods

Cool foods cause the energy within our body to sink gently downwards. A common Daoist analogy for explaining balancing the Qi within the body is the relationship between Fire and Water. Anything that expands or causes the Qi to rise would be considered to be acting like Fire, whilst anything that counters this effect would be considered Water. In part, the regulation of energetic health is understanding and managing the harmony that should exist between these two elements. Cooling foods would certainly act as the Water element within our diet. The movement of energy caused by Cooling foods is shown in Figure 23.4.

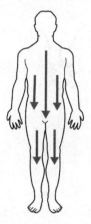

FIGURE 23.4: THE MOVEMENT OF COOL FOOD ENERGY

Cooling foods counteract the rising of Qi that takes place in the body as a result of various factors. Obviously, the most relevant to this chapter is the rising of Qi caused by an excess of Hot foods. Cooling foods can be consumed in order to help lower this rising and thus negate many of the negative effects of excess Yang qualities within the body. Qi also rises up or 'Fire is generated' through emotional stresses. The Heart is the organ through which we experience our emotional shifts and, as such, extremes of tension and excitement cause the Heart's Qi to expand outwards. Stress is obviously a major component of modern living, and so many people have an excess of rising Qi within their body. Cooling foods consumed regularly would be an easy way for the body to help regulate this rising energy. Essentially, what this means is that Cool foods can help alleviate stress and calm the mind as well as helping with a variety of health concerns.

Cooling foods are particularly important to eat on hot summer days, as they help to counter the effects that the environment has upon the body. At the same time, unless a person is already imbalanced towards being excessively Hot and Yang, they should limit their consumption of Cool foods on cold days or during the winter-time.

Cold Foods

Cold foods cause the Qi of the body to contract strongly, as shown in Figure 23.5. This contraction limits the growth and movement of Qi.

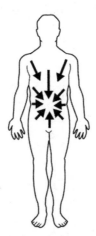

FIGURE 23.5: THE MOVEMENT OF COLD FOOD ENERGY

Contraction of Qi is almost always seen as a highly negative thing. It causes stagnation of Qi and slows the changes and evolutions that are supposed to be taking place within the body. As Qi contracts, it causes organs to go into a state of hypo-function and generally damages the Yang of the body. The body is understood to operate according to a series of 'fires', which serve as generative forces within the energetic system. This is where Daoist theory can become a little confusing! These fires are not considered negative, as in the case of the Fire generated by excessively Hot foods. For this reason, I have separated them by capitalising the fires that are considered negative when they are in extreme. The fires of the body that we wish to cultivate are primarily the lower fire and the Ming fire. These two fires are shown in Figure 23.6. There are further fires within the body, but these two are considered the most important for alchemical and internal practitioners.

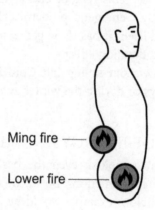

Ming fire

Lower fire

FIGURE 23.6: THE LOWER AND MING FIRES

The lower and Ming fires are essentially two expanding balls of energy, which cause energetic information to pulse outwards in smooth waves. Anybody with a degree of skill at energetic palpation can clearly feel the pulsing of the Ming fire when they place their hand around the lower back of a healthy person. These pulsing fires cause the Qi that reaches this area of the body to move through the rest of our system. The lower fire causes Jing to begin converting to Qi within the lower Dan Tien, whilst the Ming fire causes the Qi to flow along the length of the governing meridian, which flows through the centre of our back. As well as this, it also helps to govern the health of the Kidneys.

Problems come when the lower and Ming fires are 'put out' by an excess of Cold energy, a common source being consumption of an excess of Cold foods. The contracting Qi of the Cold foods causes the fires to be squeezed and essentially slowed down to a point of no longer doing their job properly. In the case of the Ming fire, this leads to Kidney and Yang deficiency, whilst in the case of the lower fire, it leads to Qi deficiency, which is generally experienced initially as lower levels of vitality and chronic fatigue. This is a particular problem for internal arts practitioners who require a nice and healthy lower fire for their training. This is why I always try and discourage my students from consuming excessively Cold foods such as ice cream or other frozen food products.

Cold foods also put a large stress upon the digestive system, according to Chinese energetic theory, as extra Qi is required to break down the food as we eat it. This is because digestion itself requires warmth – expanding Qi. This type of energy is the catalyst for the conversion of the food's energetic properties. If we don't get this warmth from the food itself, it has to be generated from inside of the body and so this has a draining effect.

It probably goes without saying but Cold foods should not be consumed on cold days or during the winter at all.

THE BALANCE OF ENERGY AND MATTER

When students begin to look at even the basics of these theories they can often find contradictions between ancient and modern understandings. An obvious example would be a food such as Sushi. According to the modern nutritional understanding of Sushi, it would be considered very healthy. It contains high levels of iodine (in the seaweed) as well as high levels of vitamins and minerals. Having selenium and omega 3 oils and being low in calories means that Sushi has become a common health food around the world. Of course, this is all true from a modern understanding, and indeed Sushi can be very healthy in this way, but from a Chinese energetic perspective it is a Cold food. This means that it can lead to a contraction of the body's Qi, which is very negative for a person's internal well-being. Sushi is, obviously, Japanese, and in ancient times they had similar understandings to the Chinese, and so consequently they countered this by only eating Sushi with accompanying warm components such as ginger or wasabi. By putting both into the body at the same time they attempted to negate the Cold effects of Sushi, but for now let us consider the example of Sushi, bereft of its warm accompaniments, as an example of the difference between energy and matter during eating. Figure 23.7 shows the process involved in eating.

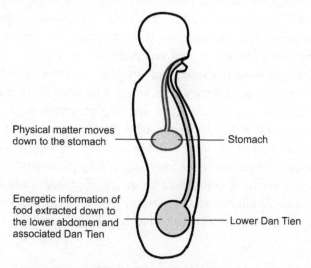

FIGURE 23.7: MATTER AND ENERGY DURING EATING

As we can see from Figure 23.7 there are two movements within the body that take place when we eat our food. The first is from the mouth to the stomach and then on into the rest of the digestive system. This is where the matter of food is processed and it is here that our body absorbs the physical nutritional elements studied in modern nutrition theory. The second pathway is from the mouth, down the front of the body, through the energetic system and into the lower abdomen, where it reacts with the lower Dan Tien. The lower Dan Tien does not absorb any of the physical matter of the food but instead receives the food's energetic information. The lower Dan Tien then processes that information and in turn creates a movement of Qi according to that energy. It basically either circulates more Qi or causes it to expand, rise, sink or contract. This is why energetically aware people will often feel the energetic movements of food taking place first in the abdomen and then the rest of the body. It is also the reason why Cold food has such a strong contractive effect upon the lower fire, which sits within the same region as the lower Dan Tien.

In the case of a food such as Sushi, the nutritional (Yin) aspect of the food will nourish the physical body via the stomach pathway, but (without the warming ginger and wasabi) its Yang component, the energetic information, will contract the body's Qi after it travels down to the lower Dan Tien region of the body. This brings me back to what I was discussing at the start of this chapter. Which conceptual model are you working to? Remember, this is not necessarily a choice as such, but rather which model have you subconsciously been working to? In the case of many internal arts practitioners, once you are past the early stages in your training you are likely to have shifted to the ancient energetic perspective. This means that your body may well be primarily working according to the Yang properties of the Sushi, the energetically contractive aspect of it. If this is the case, then the nutritional aspects of the food will be secondary with regards to your health, whilst the nature of the food's Qi will be paramount.

This is something you should be aware of in your daily life. Of course, we are all affected to some degree by both aspects of our food, but our main paradigm will control which is the most influential for us.

COOKING AND TEMPERATURES

Food itself has energetic properties in the form of the five 'temperatures', but the manner in which we prepare our food also has an influence upon its nature. This is because cooking is an energetic process in itself. In many alchemical texts the ancient Daoists use cooking as imagery to help explain what is taking place, and even the Chinese character for Qi shows the steam coming off cooking rice. How you prepare your food changes the nature of the Qi contained within it, and this in turn changes the energetic thermal nature of the food.

If we place common ways of preparing food in order, from hottest to coldest, we would have the following sequence:

- roasting (Hot)
- deep frying (Hot)
- barbecued (Hot)
- flame grilled (Hot)
- baking (Warm)

- grilled (Warm)

- frying (Warm)

- stewing (Warm)

- boiling (Neutral)

- steaming (Neutral–Cooling)

- eating raw (Cold).

This can initially seem a little strange. For example, how can boiling a food still be neutral when boiling water is hot? The answer in this lies with the fact that the 'temperatures' are actually references to the movement of energy within that food rather than a literal temperature (though of course it does play some part). Generally, Chinese cooking tends to lean towards cooking methods that are neutral or warming in nature. Roasting food is a method used rarely, and only foods with strong warming properties in themselves are considered okay to eat raw. Chinese salads are generally lightly steamed to take the edge off the Cold nature of eating raw salads.

THE ENERGETIC FLAVOURS OF CHINESE FOOD THEORY

As well as being classified according to its energetic thermal properties, food is also classified according to five energetic flavours. These flavours are Pungent, Sweet, Sour, Bitter and Salty. These flavours are essentially discussing certain energetic resonances that food has, as well as the literal flavours that we experience when we eat them. The reason this is important is because the whole of our body can be understood to resonate according to five key categories. These five key categories are also reflected in our mind, our emotions and even out into the external environment. These five classifications are known as the five elements, and these are a complete study in their own right. Chinese medicine, as well as Daoist philosophy, heavily uses the theory of the five elements; the flavours of food are one aspect of this theory. Each of the five flavours is discussed individually below.

Pungent Foods

The Pungent flavour resonates with the element of Metal, meaning that it promotes the functions of the Lungs and Large Intestine within the body. As well as this, it has an effect upon the various body systems associated with these organs, which include the skin, pores and elimination system of the body. It is understood that Pungent foods promote healthy 'distribution and circulation' or energy and fluids around the body, as well as having a stimulating effect upon our digestive processes. Many Pungent foods help to 'expel the exterior', meaning that they help to open the pores and promote the expulsion of pathogenic energies when they are close to the surface of our body. This is why ginger (a well-known Pungent food) is classically suggested for people to help energetically purge the body of a cold when it is in its early stages.

Pungent foods help to promote a healthy flow of Qi within the Lung and Large Intestine meridians, which also helps to regulate numerous aspects of our body system. A more complete list of these positive effects can be found in all in-depth Chinese medical text books.

If consumed to excess, Pungent foods will cause an unhealthy rising of the body's Qi.

Sweet Foods

The Sweet flavour resonates with the element of Earth, meaning that it promotes the functions of the Spleen and Stomach within the body. As well as this, it also has an effect upon the various body systems associated with these organs. These include the digestive system, as well as our thought processes. Sweet foods are nourishing for the body and help to provide lubrication throughout our system. Be aware of two things though. First, Sweet foods tend to be more pleasurable for many people, so consuming them in excess is always a danger. Too much of the Sweet flavour brings the opposite effect – the Spleen and Stomach are damaged and the production of the internal pathogen of Damp is inevitable. Second, Sweet foods are foods such as sweet potato, dates, honey, carrots and corn. Sugary drinks, chocolate and foods of this kind are indeed Sweet but would be considered a pathogenic version of the flavour.

Sweet foods help to promote a healthy flow of Qi in the Spleen and Stomach meridians.

If consumed to excess, Sweet foods will cause an unhealthy rising of the body's Qi.

Sour Foods

Sour foods resonate with the element of Wood, meaning that they have a close relationship with the Qi of the Liver and Gall Bladder. Foods of this flavour help to govern any excess production of fluids within the body, as well as helping with negative discharges. This means that sour foods can help with a variety of issues ranging from loose bowels through to an overproduction of Damp within the body. In this way it can be understood that the Sour, Wood food quality is helping to control the Earth element of the body.

Sour foods help to promote a healthy flow of Qi within the Liver and Gall Bladder meridians, as well as regulating energetic flow around the diaphragm. This is often missed but I feel it important to include, as many people are 'stuck' around the diaphragm region of the body.

If consumed to excess, Sour foods will cause an unhealthy sinking of the body's Qi.

Bitter Foods

Bitter foods resonate with the element of Fire, meaning that they have a close relationship with the organs of the Heart and Small Intestine. Bitter foods help the Heart and its associated organ of the Pericardium (Heart Protector in some medical traditions) to clear excess Heat from the body. This means they are foods that can help to deal with a body that is too 'Hot', providing that the food has not been prepared in such a way that it has become Hot itself! Bitter foods also help to eliminate Dampness, meaning that a person who is too sluggish and carries excess weight may well wish to up their consumption of Sour and Bitter foods in order to help tackle this issue. As well as this, they would also then have to consider the relative Yin and Yang, Cold and Hot, qualities of their internal system.

Bitter foods help with sinking Qi away from the Heart towards the lower sections of the body. For this reason, they can also help with urination and emptying of the bowels if these body functions are in a state of imbalance.

Bitter food's travel promotes a healthy flow of Qi within the Heart, Small Intestine, Pericardium and Triple Heater meridians.

If consumed to excess, Bitter foods will cause an unhealthy sinking of the body's Qi.

Salty Foods

Salty foods resonate with the element of Water and as such have a close relationship with the Kidneys and the Bladder. These foods help to free the body of stagnation, provide lubrication and promote the building of healthy Blood. They are also good foods to consume to help with the breakdown of any masses within the body. Since Salty foods affect the Kidneys, they are powerful foods to aid in an unhealthy libido or any fertility issues; an obvious example of this are oysters, which most people understand to be an aphrodisiac.

Salty foods promote a healthy flow of Qi within the Kidney and Bladder meridians.

If consumed to excess, Salty foods will cause an unhealthy sinking of the body's Qi.

According to Chinese energetic theory, a healthy diet is one that comprises a balance of the five flavours, as well as a healthy regulation of the thermal properties of the diet according to the five temperatures. Imbalance results primarily from generating an unhealthy leaning towards either being too Hot or too Cold, as well as favouring one or more of the flavours in excess. If we were to use these theories in a medical manner, a practitioner who understands what the nature of their imbalance is can adjust their food accordingly to help regulate this imbalance. In this way they are using their food as fuel and medicine – the healthiest ways to approach your diet.

A FINAL THEORY OF LIFTING AND SINKING

An interesting classical theory is based upon the idea of lifting and sinking. When I first heard this theory I was surprised by its simplicity, but it is a rule that has stuck in my mind since this time. Rules that are simple and easy to remember are the best in my opinion!

The theory states that many kinds of illness are a result of Qi either rising or sinking within the body. Note, however, that this is a separate theory and as such should not be mixed with the thermal theory of rising and sinking. We are not discussing concepts such as Hot and Cold, or Fire and Water. This is simply based upon a different understanding of Qi movement. You will find that theories like this sometimes appear to clash in Chinese medical thought. This is mainly because China is a large place with a long history. Different theories and concepts developed in different areas. Chinese medical thought has now absorbed many of these beliefs. For Western minds this can be tricky, as we tend to like a clean theory that is 100 per cent applicable all of the time. From spending a great many years travelling through China I can safely say that the Chinese do not have such issues! It does not matter to them if two theories seem to contradict each other; to the Chinese this is simply a reflection of the nature of life.

Basically, some common illnesses are caused by the sinking of Qi. These issues include loose bowels, prolapse of organs, sensations of heaviness, low energy and haemorrhoids. In contrast to this, we also have conditions caused by the rising of Qi. These are conditions such as hiccups, belching, vomiting, headaches, light-headedness and scattered thoughts.

If we wish to help regulate these conditions, then we can consume foods with the opposite properties. So, to help alleviate conditions that result from sinking Qi, we can eat food that has the quality of rising energy and vice versa.

Foods with rising Qi include vegetables and fruits that grow in trees or above the ground, as they are subject to the Qi of the air during their growth. As the air interacts with the growing vegetables it causes their energetic properties to become slightly 'floating' and, as such, if they are eaten they will help to alleviate problems caused by sinking Qi.

Food with sinking or heavy Qi are plants and vegetables that are grown below the ground. The compressing nature of the soil, combined with the damp environment they are grown in, causes them to have slightly more Yin properties. When they are consumed they help to 'anchor' imbalanced rising Qi back towards the ground, which in turn helps with 'rising Qi' conditions.

The only food that does not adhere to this theory entirely is the mushroom. Mushrooms are considered something of a 'super-food' energetically, as they contain the properties of both floating and sinking Qi. This is because they are affected by environmental Qi of both the air and the ground, as shown in Figure 23.8. This places them in the unique energetic position of helping alleviate both rising and sinking illnesses.

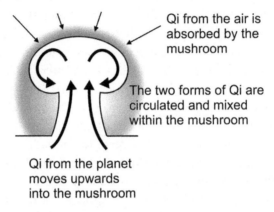

Qi from the air is absorbed by the mushroom

The two forms of Qi are circulated and mixed within the mushroom

Qi from the planet moves upwards into the mushroom

FIGURE 23.8: THE ENERGETIC PROPERTIES OF MUSHROOMS

It is interesting to note that there are whole sections of classical texts discussing mushrooms. It was considered a real art to understand how to select the best mushrooms for both your health and for psychedelic experiences via 'magic' mushrooms. For the Daoists there was a whole study of the shape and size of mushrooms, as well as the location they were grown, and even the phase of the moon they were picked during. Many of these teachings are now lost to modern practitioners, but one thing is for certain – the ancient Daoists sure were fond of mushrooms!

I hope this chapter has given a brief insight into the energetic properties of food and how the ancient Daoists viewed the subject of healthy eating. Of course, this chapter has only been an overview; many authors have explored this concept in greater detail. A quick look around online will yield a great number of books written about Chinese medical approaches to health and food. Just be sure to explore the book you find a little and make sure that it really is discussing Chinese food energetics. There are a number of books pretending to cover this subject when in actual fact they have distorted the theories by trying to mix them with modern food theories of nutrition or acid/alkaline balance. Whilst these are valid approaches to understanding healthy eating, it never works to mix theories in this way, as almost inevitably something is lost along the way.

In conclusion to the chapter, here are a few example lists of foods from different energetic categories. They should help you to get started with your study, but in order to go deeper you should find more detailed lists elsewhere.

EXAMPLE LIST OF FOODS
Energetic Food Categories
COLD FOODS
Watermelon, banana, grapefruit, pomelo, kiwi, honeydew melon, mango, papaya, seaweed, kelp, sprouts, watercress, lettuce, tomato, lemon, crab, caviar.

COOL FOODS
Millet, barley, wheat, alfalfa, buckwheat, eggplant, celery, spinach, rucola, avocado, peppermint, broccoli, cucumber, cauliflower, Chinese cabbage, amaranth, pea, mung bean, pear, apple, coconut, strawberry, orange, blueberry, bean curd, mushroom, egg white, sesame oil, cream, yogurt.

NEUTRAL FOODS
Quinoa, polenta, rye, bulgur, couscous, rice, corn, sweet potato, potato, turnip, carrot, cabbage, radish leaf, beetroot, soybean, adzuki bean, peanut, sesame seed, sunflower seed, cashew nut, pistachio nut, black sesame, sunflower seed, plum, fig, grapes, olives, white fungus, black fungus, shiitake mushroom, oyster, quail, egg yolk, beef, royal jelly honey, soybean milk, blackberry, raspberry, liquorice tea.

WARM FOODS
Leek, onion, ginger (fresh), coriander, red wine, oats, Brussels sprout, sweet pepper, pomegranate, apricot, peach, cherry, litchi, pumpkin, date, walnut, pine nut, cumin, cardamom, clove, fennel, garlic, dill

seed, parsley, basil, nutmeg, rosemary, cacao, star anise, sweet basil, vinegar, wine, vegetable oil, chicken, venison, goat milk, jasmine.

HOT FOODS

Garlic, black pepper, chilli, spicy wine, ginger (dried), cinnamon, mustard seed, lamb, refined sugar, sweet drinks, processed foods, monosodium glutamate (MSG).

Energetic Flavours

PUNGENT FOODS

Fresh ginger, onion, sweet pepper, turnip, cinnamon, tangerine peel, leek, cayenne, elderflower, scallion, fennel, green onion, garlic, celery, coriander, chilli pepper, mustard seed and wine, mint.

SWEET FOODS

Carrot, dates, sweet potato, potato, pumpkin, soybean, rice, corn, peanut, peas, apple, pear, cherry, chestnut, grapes, molasses, apricot, beet, honey, shiitake mushroom, squash, yam, almond, coconut.

SOUR FOODS

Lemon, lime, tomato, pomelo, vinegar, pickle, sauerkraut, pineapple, apple, raspberry, grape, mango, blackberry, strawberry, papaya, pear, orange, tangerine, peach, pomegranate, plum.

BITTER FOODS

Wine, vinegar, Echinacea, alfalfa, romaine lettuce, turnip, apricot seed, plum kernel, asparagus, peach kernel, bergamot, dandelion leaf, burdock leaf, yarrow, chamomile.

SALTY FOODS

Salt, seaweed, kelp, sea clams, soy sauce, miso, sea shrimps, oyster, crabs, dried mussel, cuttlefish.

A NOTE ON SUGAR

As an extra note to this chapter I should briefly mention the issue of sugar. Generally, when you look at contemporary views of Chinese food energetics, they list sugar as Neutral in nature and even as having properties of nourishing Yin and the organ of the Stomach. In contrast I have listed sugar as being Hot in nature, which essentially means that it adds to the depletion of Yin and the uprising of Yang. In this case I am discussing refined, white sugar. This is the sugar you will find in soft drinks, candy bars and, unfortunately, much of our diet these days. Certainly, when you eat out at a restaurant, many dishes have refined sugar added to them, along with MSG, another hugely Hot food substance.

In my personal opinion, refined sugar is Hot in nature and causes many problems for the body. In absolutely tiny doses refined sugar may have some kind of benefit for you or temporarily negate stress as is often listed in other sources, but I don't believe that many people use refined sugar sensibly enough for this to be the case. The amount of sugar added to many modern foods is way beyond what would be considered okay, and in my experience places it well into the unhealthy and Hot category of food.

24

ON MEDITATION AND FREEDOM

Lauren Faithfull

All ancient traditions feature some kind of meditative practice. The particular stillness that comes from sitting in quiet contemplation has always been recognised as an essential element of spiritual cultivation. Some traditions attempt to go straight to this stillness, focusing on quieting the mind and observing the breath. The Daoist tradition, recognising this as an incredibly difficult thing to do, provides us with steps that allow us to build up the space within which we can aspire to this stillness.

The first step is a prosaic one. You have an interest in Daoism, meditation, Qi Gong or some other kind of practice. You go along to a course or a class and learn some techniques, some movements and some theory. Something in the practice speaks to you, and you think that maybe this is something you'd like to carry on doing. This is your first step – eke out the time in your day to practise. Amid your job, the children, the dog, *Downton Abbey* and that lie-in you know you deserve after a busy week, you make the space to train. It's quite likely that, at the beginning, this will be an effort, a deliberate set of minutes set aside for practice. And it's quite possible that, at the beginning, you will find yourself thinking about a host of other stuff during this reserved time. That's okay. Just keep that space. You've made a start, and the act of having created space to train in the physical realm will soon lead to other types of space that can lead you deeper into your practice.

The Daoist theory of the process of creation holds that nothing can exist before consciousness. Nothing – no object, no organism, no thought, no emotion, no aspect of spirit, no action – can exist without both a Xian Tian and a Hou Tian state. Xian Tian means pre-Heaven, often called pre-natal or congenital. It is a realm of pure potential, of stillness before movement, of Wuji before Taiji. Hou Tian means post-Heaven, often called post-natal or acquired. It is manifestation; it is 'the myriad things' of the *Dao De Jing*, the world that is knowable through our five-sense reality. So, a materialist perspective might posit that life is formed when a sperm and an egg come together to form a zygote, or at the first sign of brain activity, or at the point at which the foetus is first able to survive independent of the mother. Of course, this is a complicated, and at times highly contentious, issue, but, generally speaking in this worldview, from conception, arms, legs, organs and bones come into being and gradually a human being is built. In Daoism, consciousness comes first. A spark of movement, of original intention in the realm of potential, stirs in Wuji and creates Shen, the vibrational substance of consciousness. From here, through the process of creation, the vibrational frequency of existence gets denser, through Qi and then Jing, until we have a physical expression of that vibrational frequency in the world all people experience around them daily.

Daoism is a framework that we can use to understand this world. Jing, Qi and Shen are markers within that framework that describe particular vibrational frequencies that lie behind all of existence. While these three terms all refer to a vibrational frequency, many people are only able to tune into a very limited spectrum. Broadly speaking, Jing (as discussed previously) refers to the vibrational frequency that is the closest to physical manifestation, Qi describes the vibrational frequency of the energetic realm and Shen that of the consciousness realm. For the most part, people are tuned into the Jing level. Human beings are able to contact one 'level' up or down in the Jing–Qi–Shen–Dao matrix, so when tuned into Jing, a person might get glimpses of the Qi realm – feelings of Qi running through the meridians, or getting stuck in certain areas of the body, for example. At this stage, the Shen and Dao levels are out of the range of perception. If tuned into Qi, then a person's energy body will feel as real to them as their physical body. Although still aware of the material world around, the person might feel slightly removed from it as energetic vibrational frequencies are the principal energies picked up. As Qi is also one step away from Shen, a person will be able to perceive the consciousness realm. Further training and self-cultivation can lead a person to tune fully into the consciousness realm. At this stage, the Jing level is two stages away, so perception of the physical world falls away. This is when a practitioner loses sense of the world during meditation, for example. There is still an awareness of the Qi realm, and there may be glimpses of Dao.

The relationship of change to the various vibrational frequencies is similar to the relationship of perception to the same frequencies. It's pretty difficult to tune straight into Shen, and to start touching emptiness beginning with prolonged sitting practice. I know people who get a lot of benefits from this type of meditation, where you empty your mind and just sit, but I certainly needed more guiding into it. Perhaps if you live a monastic lifestyle, or at least one with very few distractions, it might be easier, but when I first began meditating, I couldn't even focus for a few seconds. I'd settle down with the best of intentions, but soon what had happened the day before would be replaying in my head, along with plans for the weekend and a disinclination to go to work, all to a soundtrack of the most annoying song I could muster from the depths of my mind... I'd forget I was supposed to be meditating, even, dragging my mind back to my feeble attempt at nothingness after 30 minutes or more of mental chatter, feeling that I'd just wasted half an hour of precious pre-office training time. At times like that, it can be quite disheartening (especially if your training time is tight), and continuing the practice can be difficult. With Daoist alchemy, we begin by focusing on the body, on the form. This preparation can begin even before we start sitting. Stretching the body, opening the hips, strengthening the core, getting the Wuji alignments as close to perfect as you can – all of this generates huge change on the Jing (or physical) level. Change on the Jing level creates change for Qi, and that is why students often report massive improvements in mood and shifts in physical and energetic blockages after even a short-of-time training. Then, you start working on the energy body, waking the Dan Tien up and clearing things from the energy body. This sets up a virtuous cycle between energy body and physical body, as well as having a positive effect on the mind. This is the Nei Gong process that is the beginning of real internal change. We are trying to return to the source, to move from physicality to Wuji in our practice, but we have to start with physicality. Once we have prepared a strong, broad foundation, we can start to move deeper, towards space.

Once we have a daily practice, and we're certain of our sincerity in training, then we have to realise that it isn't the time spent in certain positions, or running through certain forms, that's really important. It is crucial to be completely honest with yourself at this stage. It is very easy to skip a certain aspect of training because you're telling yourself it doesn't feel right or it's not what you need at the moment, when in actual fact, it just doesn't feel *nice* and it's *exactly* what you need. It can be difficult to differentiate, but it's important to analyse your attitudes to the training and recognise any reactions that are born of laziness, fear or discomfort (strangely enough, it's often core work and the more difficult Dao Yin exercises that people feel the most significant aversion to!). Having assessed your motives and confirmed that they are genuine, it is useful to begin considering the concept of Wei Wu Wei (為無為) in your training. Wei Wu Wei doesn't mean non-doing, sitting on the sofa, commenting on internet forums whilst holding a copy of the *Dao De Jing* and feeling like a Daoist. It means not governing the training. It's knowing when you are ready to let go of the rigidity of daily timetables and move from that form to a more formless type of practice. Instead of creating space just to make time for training, we begin to create a space to allow a process of change to take place, and we allow that change to come from the realm of potential. We can spend hours making shapes, but we have to change our mind, too. Through diligent preparation of the body, the mind will have begun to open up and calm. The training then begins to take place in the space that we have created. The training is not controlled: it is allowed to happen. It is at this stage that training just becomes 'something you do'. It's no longer a struggle to fit the hours in, and you don't feel as if you need to bend everything in your life to fit what you are doing – it just fits by itself. This isn't by virtue of more time or a change in circumstances; it's a change inside. We don't feel the need to convert anyone to the joys of what we're doing, because we understand that what we're doing is a strange, beautiful alchemy integral to *our* lives, but that perhaps won't suit everyone. We begin to touch on what it might mean to let the congenital nature start to emerge through the multiple layers of the acquired mind. This applies to all arts, but is particularly true of Nei Dan. At the beginning (and, let's be clear, the beginning lasts for years), you're sitting there, thinking about everything. If I can even glimpse calmness of mind, let alone stillness, for a few minutes out of an hour, I feel as if I'm doing really well. But this is okay – it feels as if I am slowly building a practice that might allow me to touch stillness, and I think that touching stillness allows us to touch freedom.

There is a lot of discussion presently about freedom – what it is, to whom it should apply and when it should be restricted. In general, freedom is said to be sacred, a universal right of all human beings. In practice, it is a little more complicated. From the moment we begin to process the world around us, we are bombarded by messages that instil fear in us and take away space for contemplation and reflection. Life becomes a series of challenges and distractions from those challenges. The search for any sense of deeper meaning is lost in the newspapers, detailing death and destruction all over the planet. The adverts, un-ignorable in their attempt to sell you youth, beauty and success. The reminder that, at 15 years old, you needed to think ahead, study hard, pass your exams. In spite of this, we are constantly reminded that our freedom is under attack. From terrorists who want to impose alien systems of law upon us. From governments who want to micromanage our lives and everything in it. From immigrants who steal our jobs and alter the lie of our cultural landscape. But what are these freedoms? Are they dependent upon allowing those with certain job titles unfettered access to your phone calls and emails? Is freedom being allowed to own as many guns as you like, in a country like America, where there are over 81,000 non-fatal and over 31,000 fatal gun-related incidents per year?[1] Is the world a better place if you have the right to offend swathes of people who believe in a god different from yours, or in any god, or no god at all? Or if you only hear your own language spoken on the streets when you go out to buy your bread and eggs? The longer I spend studying the internal arts, the more convinced I become that the whole edifice is built on a foundation of fear, and that the key to true freedom is vanquishing these fears. I believe that to do this we need space that we can slowly build in our life through practice, which makes meditation a strange and powerful kind of rebellion. However, I don't think that space alone is the solution to the world's ills. Space gives us freedom; what we do within it is our own personal cultivation. This is why you can meet practitioners – sometimes they are teachers

1   Cornell, D. G. (2014) 'Gun violence and mass shootings – myths, facts and solutions.' *The Washington Post*, 11 June. Available at www.washingtonpost.com/ news/the-watch/wp/2014/06/11/gun-violence-and-mass-shootings-myths-facts-and-solutions, accessed on 23 April 2016.

with pretty sizeable followings – who are driven by base desires and materialist motives. People who have dedicated their lives to practice, perhaps even become highly skilled, using their knowledge to make as much money as possible, sexually exploit their students or simply just revel in the power and status afforded by being perceived as an authority in spiritual matters. Within our space, we're free to be as unethical, immoral or unpleasant as we wish to be; our process of cultivation should involve questioning why we feel the need to do certain things and act in certain ways. Considering how you treat and react to others does not mean restricting freedom – there are numerous writers who proudly state that nothing and no one will stop them from saying whatever they want, implying that being allowed to call immigrants 'cockroaches' is the best that humanity can strive to offer in its quest for freedom.[2] Instead, it means constantly analysing your own actions and trying to understand your motives. Freedom shouldn't be the liberty to offend, to hurt, to belittle. It should be disentanglement from the acquired mind (or the ego) that is constantly trying to promote self-interest, to compete, to feel superior and safe in its individuality. We don't want to get rid of the acquired mind, because we need it to converse and travel and work and play. However, we don't want to be a slave to it. If we can begin to still the mind within our space, we can quiet the acquired mind to give congenital nature the floor, and congenital nature won't want to close borders, acquire riches or create hateful divisiveness between people. It doesn't even have a concept of what prejudice, nationality or wealth mean.

David Foster Wallace, for a commencement speech at a US college in 2005, spoke beautifully about how we can choose how to think, and how to find meaning in life. He said:

> ...in the day-to-day trenches of adult life, there is actually no such thing as atheism. There is no such thing as not worshipping. Everybody worships. The only choice we get is what to worship. And the compelling reason for maybe choosing some sort of god or spiritual-type thing to worship – be it JC or Allah, be it YHWH

2　ITV (2015) 'Katie Hopkins compares migrants to "cockroaches" and suggests using gunships to stop them crossing the Mediterranean.' *ITV News*, 18 April. Available at www.itv.com/news/2015-04-18/katie-hopkins-compares-migrants-to-cockroaches-and-suggests-using-gunships-to-stop-them-crossing-the-mediterranean, accessed on 23 April 2016.

or the Wiccan Mother Goddess, or the Four Noble Truths, or some inviolable set of ethical principles – is that pretty much anything else you worship will eat you alive. If you worship money and things, if they are where you tap real meaning in life, then you will never have enough, never feel you have enough. It's the truth. Worship your body and beauty and sexual allure and you will always feel ugly. And when time and age start showing, you will die a million deaths before they finally grieve you. On one level, we all know this stuff already. It's been codified as myths, proverbs, clichés, epigrams, parables; the skeleton of every great story. The whole trick is keeping the truth up front in daily consciousness.

Worship power, you will end up feeling weak and afraid, and you will need ever more power over others to numb you to your own fear. Worship your intellect, being seen as smart, you will end up feeling stupid, a fraud, always on the verge of being found out. But the insidious thing about these forms of worship is not that they're evil or sinful, it's that they're unconscious. They are default settings.[3]

I actually come back to this speech time and time again, as it serves as an eloquent reminder of what I would like to do within the space that I'm trying to create. With that in mind, I think that perhaps, ultimately, freedom is being able to choose how to best use the acquired mind to navigate life without feeling the need to marginalise, deprecate or oppress others who are themselves just trying to figure out their path.

---

3   The Economist, 'David Foster Wallace, in his own words.' *The Economist 1843*, 19 September. Available at www.1843magazine.com/story/david-foster-wallace-in-his-own-words, accessed on 23 April 2016.

25

THE HUN AND SYMBOLISM

Donna Pinker

The Hun (魂) is our ethereal soul. It expresses reality by employing the creative, the symbolic, the metaphorical and the poetic. Its opposite is the Po (魄), our corporeal soul. We can interpret reality through our Po or through our Hun.

Within the West, there exists an over-tendency to interpret reality through the limiting perception of the Po. The Po employs our five senses and analytical mind. It has a propensity to separate, dissect, segregate and categorise the world. The Po speaks in language. The Po is corporeal and ceases at the time of death. Its faculties are the five senses, the emotions, personality, mind and the ego, which also cease when the physical body perishes. These faculties all limit and reduce data received from the world into manageable packets.

In contrast, the Hun connects to the unlimited. It can directly intuit a meaning of a concept, and does so through less restrictive language such as a symbol, a metaphor, an allegory, poetry or art. The Hun has no limits and accesses information directly, without spatial or temporal context, allowing a 'knowing'.

In order to follow the Daoist path we need to balance our Po and Hun souls; our emotions and our nature. This entails familiarising ourselves with our own nature, our Hun souls. Table 25.1 lists qualities of the Hun and the Po souls.

Table 25.1: Qualities of the Hun and the Po Souls

Hun	Po
Mythical	Analytic
Non-linear	Linear
Integrative	Analytic
Pictograph writing	Phonetic language
Relationships between objects, event and experiences	Deductions
Coincidence of connections	Isolated incidents
Patterns	Cause and effect
Totality	Separation
Holistic	Predictive
Creation manifests in patterns and cycles	Creator God
Poetry	Logical
Symbols	Directed thought
Creativity	A single objective
Dreams	Focused, pinpointed
Energetic system	Anatomy and physiology
Meridians	Organs
Qi	Surgery

The Western scientific mindset tends to deduce, separate and categorise. Its analytic process focuses on cause and effect, whereas Eastern metaphysical systems operate with totalities. Eastern philosophies assert that no single part can be understood, except in its relationship within the whole. Overall patterns, rather than linear cause-and-effect relationships, are the prime factor in understanding. This fundamental difference in understanding is reflected in the metaphysical systems found in the West and the East. The Western tradition proliferated religious beliefs in a divine being who created the manifest universe at a specific time. The Buddhist and Daoist traditions view creation as continuously manifesting in patterns and cycles within the world everywhere.

The two divergent logics are also reflected within medical systems. The West isolates specific diseased areas in the body, whereas the East deals with a person's totality. This is why it is so important in the West not to allow the Western medical tradition to reduce Chinese medicine to a cause-and-effect diagnostic treatment.

According to Chinese mythology, language was a gift from the gods in prehistoric times. The Chinese characters were regarded as nets in which the light of spirit could be gathered. I like this notion, because writing in pictographs is richer and more multidimensional than our own sentence-based alphabetic writing. Pictographs are immediately perceived wholes that unify a host of related impressions and ideas. Each character is a symbol. Take the character for the sun, which is shown in Figure 25.1. This is the ancient version of the character for sun.

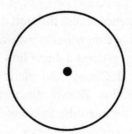

FIGURE 25.1: Ri – Sun

This symbol for sun not only says 'sun', it also combines multiple impressions of the sun, including roundness and centrality, and also means day. A character or symbol condenses many layers of meaning and related expressions. They reflect universal archetypes. Two or more characters can be combined to portray new meaning. For example, sun and moon together can be translated as brightness. Yet, inherent in the combined character is so much more than our English word 'bright'. Images of a dazzling shiny sun in a perfect sky, or a perfect full-shining white moon, are conjured in the imagination. This is shown in Figure 25.2 – the character 'Ming'.

Pictographs or symbols are powerful motifs for conjuring within us the archetypal meaning. The symbol creates a resonance that vibrates through time and space to affect our experience on subtle levels. Asiatic people who translate their written word in this manner are in contact with their Hun soul more than their Western counterparts.

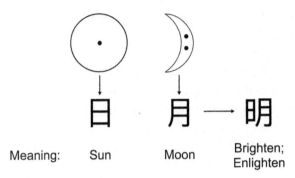

| Meaning: | Sun | Moon | Brighten; Enlighten |

FIGURE 25.2: MING – BRIGHT

The Po soul employs the five senses and controls the five emotions of the Wu Xing (五行), and hence, the Po controls the classical meridians. The Hun soul controls our essential nature, and hence, our congenital meridians. The Po's experience is limited by the transient sense faculties. To experience reality through the Hun soul is therefore to experience through the congenital meridians and energetic system. The congenital meridians process a direct link to the energies of Earth and Heaven. Our central Chong Mai meridian acts as an antenna conducting the information drawn down from Heaven. Man is positioned as a conduit between the forces of Heaven and Earth.

The Chong Mai extends outside our physical bodies, and this energetic field feeds information back to us, which is sensed intuitively, via our energetic system. The Daoist practice of Shen Gong (神功) utilises this facility, allowing us to sense the energies within nature and other people. The practice of Shen Gong allows us to connect with a tree and feel its Wood energy rising and pushing out. Linking our energy systems to the energy of nature gives us direct energetic experience. For example, a blossoming flower may create an expansive radiance within the middle Dan Tien, as it is an expression of Fire energy.

Whilst connecting to energies in this manner we can also receive relevant information that speaks in the language of symbols and metaphors. Our rationalistic Po soul will see a tree with our eyes, possibly smell it with our nose and hear the wind blow through its leaves. The Po will possibly categorise it by giving it a name, or judging its size against another, or identify its leaf shape. On the other hand, our Hun soul will read the tree in symbols that speak to us on a more personal level.

He who sees the infinite in all things sees God.
He who sees the ratio sees himself only.

'There is No Natural Religion', William Blake

Mandalas, sacred symbolism, emblems, talismans, poetry and art are often utilised in religious and esoteric philosophies. This is sometimes to hide information, but invariably it is also because far more information can be conveyed than through the rationalistic, narrowly defined nature of the written word. Daoism makes use of several symbolic images to portray its cosmological metaphysics. The Yin/Yang divides the universe into two forces. The five phases of the Wu Xing have their elemental forces and cycles. The Chinese calendar represents seasonal and planetary rhythms and patterns with totemic animals. The *Yi Jing* encompasses a detailed outline of alchemical timing and provides a diagrammatic blueprint of cosmology and alchemy. Figure 25.3 shows the Wu Xing chart.

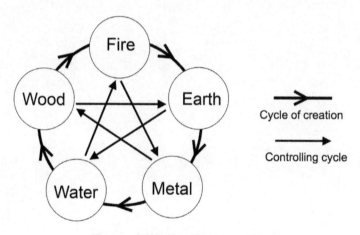

FIGURE 25.3: THE WU XING CHART

The Wu Xing embodies far more than at first appears. The colour, flavour, direction, season, tone, smell, emotion and force are grouped together, because they each represent the same vibration in reality, but they are perceived by the senses in a different form. The symbolic representation allows for a more profound understanding of reality on a more ephemeral level than a linguistic description could achieve through the engagement of Po cognition. For this reason, knowledge is transmitted to spiritual students via the use of the abstract. Within alchemy, the symbol is not only an approximate description of inward processes, it is also a revelation, giving us profound insight.

> Things in our world today are conceptualised as nothing more than 'objects' by our language and rational perspective. Although this makes it simpler to deal with the world around us, it has stifled the changeable or 'living aspect' in everything. (Masunaga 1987)

BIBLIOGRAPHY

Burckhardt, T. (2006) *Alchemy: Science of the Cosmos, Science of the Soul.* Louisville: Fons Vitae.

Dechar, L. E. (2006) *Five Spirits.* New York: Lantern Books.

Masunaga, S. (1987) *Zen Imagery Exercises: Meridian Exercises for Wholesome Living.* Tokyo: Japan Publications.

Reichstein, G. (1998) *Wood Becomes Water.* New York: Kodansha International.

26

THE REAL PURPOSE OF TRAINING

Tino Faithfull

Look —
You won't see it.
Listen —
You won't hear it.
Use it —
You will never use it up.

Dao De Jing (Verse 35)

Most animals seem to function primarily on instinct. Deep intellectual or philosophical reflection (as we understand it, at least) does not appear to be part of their experience. Within the wide animal kingdom, humans stand out through their obsessive need to intellectualise and analyse everything. Whether this is an effect of nature or nurture (or both (or neither)), I guess ultimately it doesn't really matter.

As human individuals, we ask ourselves many questions – most of the time pointless questions... But we can't help it, it seems. Humans are often drawn towards grand metaphysical questions.

- 'Why are we here?'

- 'Why are we alive rather than dead?'

- 'What is the meaning of life?'

At other times, more specific or pragmatic questions will arise.

- 'Why do we have to work?'

- 'What is the purpose of money?'

- 'Why are we ruled by banks, corporations and royal families?'

- 'Why am I a useless, depressed idiot?'

And so on…

Of course, people's personalities differ widely. Some of us are naturally outgoing and find it relatively easy to deal with life without having to look into things too deeply. Others will be more prone to questioning everything; these are usually the more introverted people. In a talk she gave a few years ago, American writer Susan Cain suggested that our modern societies are generally geared towards extroverts. As a result, Cain pointed out, more introverted people are rarely to be seen in the public arena. Introverts are often natural thinkers; because of this particular disposition, they are in a privileged position to question the status quo. This is why they should play an important role in all aspects of public life, Cain argues. I recommend you check out her talk, as it's both insightful and inspiring.[1]

If our societies are geared towards extroverts, as Cain thinks, this is definitely not something to be celebrated. Rather, this bias indicates a deep imbalance in the institutions that structure our lives. On the other hand, excessive thinking and questioning can cause equally problematic imbalances. Ideally, we should find the right balance in all things – this is what ancient spiritual traditions like Daoism advocated. In our modern languages, we use terms like 'introvert' and 'extrovert'. Like most of the words we use, these idioms carry a lot of cultural baggage and so they can mean different things. Daoism is founded on the understanding that language is a fundamentally treacherous institution. This is made clear in the very first line of the *Dao De Jing* (Verse 1): 'The Dao that can be spoken of is not the eternal Dao.' The same idea appears in Zhuangzi's ramblings:

> The purpose of words is to convey ideas. When the ideas are grasped, the words are forgotten. Where can I find a man who has forgotten words? He is the one I would like to talk to.[2]

1   Cain, S. (2012) 'The Power of Introverts.' Available at: www.ted.com/talks/susan_cain_the_power_of_introverts, accessed on 23 April 2016. In this talk, Cain draws from Carl Jung's theory of introvert and extrovert personalities.

2   Merton, T. (2004) 'Means and Ends.' In *The Way of Chuang Tzu*. Boston and London: Shambhala, p.179.

In order to avoid the common pitfalls of language, Daoism uses neutral terms. Instead of using words like 'introvert' and 'extrovert', it refers to Yin or Yang character traits.

Most people usually have a leaning towards either Yin or Yang character traits. From a Daoist perspective, those traits are considered imbalances that need to be addressed within our work of cultivation. Yin people might feel an affinity with the more introspective practices (e.g. Qi Gong or meditation), while Yang people may be drawn towards more physically based activities (e.g. external martial arts). Yin people will generally ask themselves too many questions, while Yang people might lack self-reflection. Obviously, these two categories are incredibly reductive as there are many shades of grey between the two extremes of Yin and Yang. The human psyche is intricate and full of subtleties; as such, it cannot be reduced to a set of opposites. Yin and Yang are only tools that can help us reflect on more abstract aspects of life. Once we have a basic understanding of a given model, we can depart from it. Daoism talks about moving from the realm of form to the realm of the formless.

Ideally, there should be a balance between Yin and Yang in all of us. When we start training, major imbalances in our character progressively fade away; as a result, we are healthy and content. The noise of the world becomes irrelevant – all of it. The pervy media, the obscene adverts, the glamorisation of our basest desires everywhere... Those things suddenly appear for what they are: ridiculous and pointless. We stop operating in a hyper-Yang mental mode. On the other hand, the Yin aspect of our psyche is also kept in check as we stop asking ourselves too many irrelevant questions. If we were prone to excessive introspection, this tendency should start to disappear too.

Living in a realm of constant introspection and self-questioning can create mental stagnation and prevent us from seeing what is really important in life. However, the opposite mindset can be equally harmful. A lack of reflection and self-analysis will hinder your development as an individual. As a result, your potential for growth in the internal arts will be very limited. In order to reach mental balance, we need equal amounts of Yin and Yang in our personality.

When it comes to training, questions will inevitably arise along the way. Because of their complex nature, the internal arts will stimulate your mind in an intense way (providing you have chosen to engage with this training for many years). This is a healthy process that should be embraced. As we start developing through our practice, we should become naturally more discerning. It is hoped that we can begin to see things as they really are, especially when it comes to our own thought patterns. It should become easier to identify an irrelevant question when it pops into our mind – and so we should be able to dismiss it as such.

Of course, not all questions are pointless. There are questions that will keep popping up in your head throughout the years. Sometimes it will feel as if the answer should be obvious, and yet that answer (supposing there is one) will keep eluding you. Such questions are usually the ones that need to be considered carefully.

In my case, there is one particular question that has come up time and again throughout the years…

WHY DO I TRAIN?

Why do we train, indeed? Maybe this is a trivial question. Our expectations (or lack thereof) will inevitably affect the direction that our art will take. Expectations are a form of intention – and intention is the driving force behind everything. You might think: 'I train so I can be healthy again.' Or you might tell your friends: 'I train because I want to be enlightened.' You could also be interested in developing control over other people (although you might not be aware of it). These are very different types of intentions that will take you down different alleys in life.

The number of possible paths for your mind to take is virtually limitless. This is why we must consider our intentions with care. There must always be a degree of self-analysis along our study of the internal arts. Most spiritual or religious traditions have some sort of ethical code of conduct – Christian commandments and Buddhist precepts being two obvious examples. Unlike those systems, Daoism has no predetermined set of moral values for its students to follow. This is why we must always question our motives and intentions alongside our training.

The Daoist internal arts have the potential to alter completely your perception of reality. If practised diligently, they will shift the way you look at yourself and the world around you. However, in order to harness the full potential of those arts, we must develop the right kind of intention, as our practice will magnify our intention. If your intention is warped, the training will turn you into a warped person; it is a double-edged sword that must be wielded with care.

When I started training in the internal arts, I had very little sense of why I was training – although I had a distinct feeling that something had been amiss. It is quite common for people to take up training as a result of challenging personal circumstances such as depression, stress, anxiety or illness (to name but a few). Underlying your mental state, there might also be a diffuse sense of unease with modern life – a feeling that something is not quite right. This was definitely true in my case. For most of my pre-training life, I had felt a general sense of inadequacy and a longing for something radically different. Many people are in this situation. Unfortunately, not everybody has the chance to encounter a system that will give them the right tools to channel their feelings of frustration and inadequacy so they can be turned into something less destructive.

The study of the Daoist arts can be divided into three broad categories: the martial arts, the medical arts and the spiritual arts. There are normally specific reasons that lead people to gravitate towards particular systems of cultivation; those reasons are almost always the same, so they can be listed very easily. Thus, it is common for people to start studying the martial arts in order to up their confidence. The medical arts will often attract people who are either ill or obsessed with health. People who lack a sense of purpose or look for meaning in life may turn to the spiritual arts. I'm guessing the vast majority of people studying the internal arts will fall into one of those categories. In my opinion, becoming more confident and healthy or finding a higher purpose are all valid reasons for starting to train in the internal arts. In the early stages these reasons are your fuel; they will provide you with the necessary drive to keep on training for the following years.

I'm afraid it's difficult to talk about the internal arts in general without making sweeping statements. I'm fully aware that you may not fit any of the above-mentioned categories. Putting these thoughts down on paper is also a way for me to develop – not only as a teacher, but also as a student of the Daoist arts. In those arts, you remain a student for life.

Many years ago, my teacher took me by surprise when he asked me, in the middle of an unrelated conversation 'So...why do you train?' It took me a few seconds to answer him, as honestly as I could. Strangely, my answer was: 'I don't know.' I had no idea why I was training...

I'd already trained for a while when my teacher came up with that question. By then, I had achieved most of the basic goals that people often set themselves when they start training in the internal arts. By this, I do not mean enlightenment or superpowers; I mean things like overall health, balance and confidence. As for the sense of purpose, it became firmly established the moment I started training. Let's say that, after a few years of consistent training, the groundwork had been laid. Once this has been done, several options open up to us. We can be content with what has been achieved or we can decide to move further down the rabbit hole. For many people, this is a critical stage. If you are honest with yourself, then this is when you may encounter your real motives (and in a way your real self).

Once we have achieved a state of relative balance, the real work of internal development can begin. If we have been ill for many years, then the only thing we can think about (understandably) is being healthy. If we have had issues with confidence for most of our life, we probably wish to get over that crippling situation. If we have lacked a sense of purpose or failed to see any meaning in life, we may be determined to change. It is hoped that the training will have provided us with all these things, supposing the system of cultivation we are studying is both authentic and complete.

This is all good; we are now healthy, balanced human individuals.

There might be other reasons why we train though – let's call them 'ulterior motives'. As long as we are focused on meeting some of our most basic needs (mentioned above), those ulterior motives remain hidden. Common ulterior motives for training in the internal arts are power, control, fame, sexual gratification and money. If we're honest with ourselves, these motives will surface as soon as the 'basic needs' part of the training is done. If we wish to get anywhere with our work of cultivation, we must be bluntly honest with ourselves. This is why we should always probe our reasons for training.

Facing our ulterior motives can be a painful experience, but it will also help us to keep growing in our art. In order to develop, we must 'chew bitter' (a classical saying); it is a difficult and necessary stage in our training. However, this is only another stage in our development, not an end in itself – no more than achieving health is an end from the perspective of the Daoist arts. By definition, there are always more stages ahead of us anyway. Facing our ulterior motives is not the ultimate reason why we train; thank god for that!

So what is the real purpose of training? I do not know, and I do not particularly feel that there needs to be a specific answer to that question. The deeper I go in my own training, the less I know why I am doing it. For the time being, I am quite happy saying that I train because I train. I might change my mind in the future though; in which case, I shall write a follow-up to this chapter!

27

NATURE'S MEDICINE
Seb Smith

When peace comes at last to those who wrestle with temptation,
when the light comes at last into the mind given to contemplation…
it always comes with just one happy realization: 'I need do nothing.'
(*A Course in Miracles*, Chapter 18.VII 5 (7))

One of the side effects of our modern, technology-driven lifestyle is
that we are being continually bombarded with information. Especially
since the relatively recent advent of the smartphone, there is hardly a
minute in the day when we are not able to saturate our minds with
audio-visual stimulation and most knowledge is accessible from
anywhere at any time. This is not necessarily a bad thing, but it does
make it difficult to reach that state of inner quietude that is normally
considered a requisite for many spiritual disciplines.

The ideal state is to be able to make use of the vast quantity
of information available nowadays without being addicted to it or
dependent on it. Certain appealing character traits such as patience,
mental clarity and the ability to concentrate are slowly being displaced
and are becoming more unnecessary when the answers to many
questions are but a click away and when certain desires can be fulfilled
in an instant. There is nothing wrong with this either if what you want
from life is amply provided by modern conveniences.

We are living in an age of plenty (however it may be distributed),
and the paradigm we are subscribed to suggests that health and joy
are by-products of the ever-increasing upward climb towards having
more. More ownership of possessions, more technology, more drugs,
more money, etc. Any loss of peace or any sign of faltering mental
or physical health are presumed to be cured by having more of
something. So if you become dissatisfied in some way when living
by the value system that you are taught by society, it is automatic for

most of us to revert back to the accumulative behaviour patterns that may in fact have been the cause of 'dis-ease' in the first place. I think it is an amusing irony that often the best thing we can do for ourselves is nothing, but no one even seems to be able to manage that.

Fasting is becoming an ever more popular health intervention. Eating nothing (or nearly nothing) is becoming recognised as having numerous health benefits and is no longer considered the domain of quacks and ascetics. Fasting the mind through meditation is also happily on the rise. Later Daoist practices embrace this extreme view and entirely disconnect the mind from the body, which also produces interesting results...

Along this train of thought is my belief that all organisms have inherent self-righting mechanisms and are able to adjust and correct themselves on all levels – psychologically, physically and emotionally. I think these mechanisms are continually active, but it is only when we learn to suspend the normal hubbub of mental and physical activity that they gain the necessary momentum to undo the harmful effects of our lifestyles. I will briefly look at how this occurs in man according to Daoist theory, look at the application of this principle in society, relationships and the individual, and finally look at the implications this has for Daoist meditation (Nei Dan) practice.

For many things, people will commonly search for a quick fix. This is fairly easy within the spheres of knowledge and entertainment, as previously discussed, but for more worthwhile achievements in life one has to be ready to put in the hours. Whether you want to lose weight, get fit or learn a new skill, for example, a degree of effort is involved. Osho very aptly (and without saying 'fuck') put it thus:

> Instant coffee is possible, but instant God is not possible, so if one insists that 'I would only like that which is instantly possible', then [one will only] have coffee and no God. Then life becomes trivial, mundane; and it is a sacrilege to destroy life in small things. (Osho, *Snap Your Fingers, Slap Your Face and Wake Up!*)

So change, especially positive change and particularly of the physical body, is bound to take time and effort. I venture that it takes around two weeks at the minimum to begin to notice changes in your body if you exercise every day. By then you may become aware of how your muscles begin to thicken and your heart beats more comfortably as you push yourself further. The body is an object existing within space-time, so, intuitively, changes within the 'space' of your body will have to take time.

Interestingly, however, as consciousness exists outside the limits of space and time, it is possible for huge shifts to occur in your psychological makeup in an instant. I recall a story on this point that I found both fascinating and inspiring. On a Dao Yin course many years ago, we received a valuable mini-talk midway through one of the classes. We were being taught how to purge stagnant information from the meridian system using these Dao Yin exercises, many of which involve reverse breathing and pushing out with a strong focus – this is what we associate with Dao Yin. The secret, however, is that for these practices to work at all you need two ingredients. The first is the exercise itself, including the breathing, posture and intention. The second and most important is the willingness to let go of the trauma or residual illness that you are trying to clear. Without this you will ultimately go nowhere with these types of exercise. We were taught that if you can completely let go of all your attachment and identification with past emotional traumas, and if no part of you wants to remain sick in some way, then in the blink of an eye all of the stagnation within the energy body will vanish. The process of clearing the energy body, which conservatively takes around three years, can be done in a heartbeat. For the outstandingly rare individuals who can make this mental switch, the process takes no time and no effort at all.

I find it interesting to note that it is when the body and mind are in quiescent states that a lot of the rejuvenating effects of the Daoist arts appear. At the grossest level we are familiar with the fact that when we enter a fast and rest the digestive system then the body begins to 'detoxify' itself. Naturally, digestion should be an energy-liberating process rather than an energy-consuming process overall. Unfortunately, for most people the combination, quality and quantity of what we eat is quite far removed from what our bodies need. As a result, the simple act of digesting a meal becomes laborious and it is considered common if not entirely normal to feel bloated and tired after a meal – what some may call 'satisfaction'. Rather than supporting the functions of the body, our diet depletes and scatters the energy of our organs, particularly that of the Spleen. Fasting, then, negates the loss of energy that our digestion usually entails, and our organs then turn their attention to purifying the body rather than trying to extract the pure fraction of what we eat.

Similarly, when we meditate we shut off the senses and allow our continuous mental chatter to die down, which gradually gives the mind space to relax. When the 'Yi' or our 'intention' – the spiritual facet of the Earth element – begins to settle, our attention is not absorbed in external events or inwardly on the senses. Traditionally, the Earth element is said to sit at the centre of the other four elements (Fire, Metal, Water and Wood), so that when you disengage the Yi from being aware of anything outwardly or inwardly, it performs its function of centralising the other four facets of your spirit (Shen, Po, Zhi, Hun) to bring them back into harmony. This principle is shown in Figure 27.1.

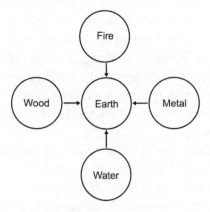

FIGURE 27.1: THE CENTRALISATION OF THE FIVE ELEMENTS

The same principle also applies to the common Qi Gong phenomenon of spontaneous energetic movement. When you are practising Qi Gong, for example in the Wuji posture, you rest your mind in the area of the lower Dan Tien and direct your breathing to that area, approximately behind your navel. The combination of your intention, breath and centre of gravity all combining in that one area starts to stimulate and awaken the Dan Tien, during which it will begin to awaken and shakily move Qi through the meridian system, which can generate movements of the physical body. This is known as Zi Fa Gong (自發功) and is a process that, once started, will continue by itself without any intervention from the mind, clearing blockages and opening up the body from within.

As we can see from the examples of fasting the body, fasting the mind and Zi Fa Gong (once the Dan Tien is at least starting to rotate and activate), a lot of the processes by which the body and mind rebalance are done without us consciously directing them; they unfold naturally if we provide the still conditions necessary for them to arise spontaneously. This is alluded to in the *Dao De Jing* (translated by Damo Mitchell) in the very potent 15th verse, the end of which says:

> Common men have muddied their water... Who can sit in quietude and allow the waters to clear? Clearing the waters leads to a new and spontaneous movement. Understand what it is to remain empty, Never fill, never age, Thus we will escape the boundaries of birth and death.

Dao De Jing (Verse 15)

Throughout the course of our lives we unwittingly accrue layers on the surface of our Heart-Mind, which veils our true consciousness and distorts both our perception of the world and the way that we outwardly express ourselves and engage with other people. This happens to us all and is unfortunately a self-perpetuating cycle that leads people into further ignorance and delusion. Therefore, in certain stages of our practice, we cut out the mind and its damaging influence on our state of being.

It becomes clear after a while that it is the interaction of the mind with the physical and energy bodies that is the greatest cause of ill health and suffering on the individual level, and that only by disconnecting the mind from the body can we begin to heal ourselves effectively. Some serious practitioners took this principle to the extreme of dissolving the mind entirely. This results in a complete lack of intellect and no information-processing ability on the physical plane of life. Whilst able to reach deep states of meditation and inner illumination, these people cannot function – to the extent they have to be led around by the hand and fed as you would do for an infant. A more sensible aim perhaps is to clear the mind of destructive attachments and habits while maintaining the ability to function amongst society.

Daoism believes in being concise. It is a no-frills guide to awakening in the most efficient manner possible. As such, it has represented the human mind simply as being in one of two states, each of which has a corresponding trigram. Humans are said to exist between the macrocosmic powers of Heaven and Earth, which are respectively Yang (Heaven) and Yin (Earth). Figure 27.2 shows the symbolic representations of these two poles.

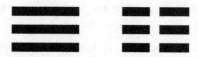

FIGURE 27.2: HEAVEN AND EARTH

These trigrams represent the pure Yang and pure Yin vibration frequencies that energetically characterise these forces that envelop us in the macrocosmic environment. In generating the symbol for man (Ren) the above trigrams are condensed into one Yang (solid) line above and one Yin (broken) line below. As such, you get the symbol shown in Figure 27.3, with the symbol for man being the division of heaven into earth.

FIGURE 27.3: HEAVEN, MAN AND HUMANITY

This is the origin for the symbol for humanity, but of course this is not a trigram. With a Yang line on top and a Yin line underneath, there are obviously two potential trigrams; the middle line can be either Yin or Yang. Therefore, the human mind is characterised either by the Wind or the Mountain trigram, as shown in Figure 27.4.

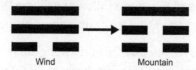

Wind   Mountain

FIGURE 27.4: WIND AND MOUNTAIN

When our mind reflects the Wind trigram, we have a representation of the mind in a more temperamental state that is unstable and prone to change. The trigram is Yin beneath two Yang lines – this is top heavy and is liable to become unsettled easily; the Yin line destabilises the solidity above it.

When the middle line, which represents man, is Yin, as in the Mountain trigram, we get the symbol that demonstrates stillness and stability – the mind in a calmer and less cluttered state.

It is fascinating to note that the two trigrams that represent the states of mankind simultaneously demonstrate the frequency of the mental activity of the persons as well as showing the relationship between humanity and the environmental powers of Heaven and Earth. It is an important Daoist principle that the internal state of a person and her relationship to her environment are linked and are in a sense one and the same thing. This is one of the founding principles of Feng Shui; if there were no correlation between the energetic frequencies within the body and the energetic frequencies outside the body then disciplines such as this and astrology would be useless to us and would not exist within the pragmatic Daoist sects.

The stability that is represented by the Mountain trigram can partly be reached by fasting of mind and body. However, at a more advanced level the deeper symbolic meaning is regarding the relationship between the energy system of a practitioner and the forces of Heaven and Earth. What is meant is that when a practitioner can reach the stage of 'energetic emptiness' where the meridian system is fully opened and devoid of any blockages, the subtle frequencies of the environment can be reeled in via the thrusting meridian (Chong Mai) through the rotation of the lower Dan Tien and circulated round the body. This balances Yin and Yang within the body at a high level and gives rise to profound levels of health and mental clarity. Thoughts and actions are influenced by the shifting energies of the cosmos, and have a greater sense of purpose than when we are governed by the mundane whims of the ego. It is at this level that one is able to give himself over to the powers of Heaven and Earth and follow the divine Will of Heaven. My favourite verse from the *Dao De Jing* describes this beautifully:

> Everlasting Heaven, eternal Earth, Existing forever, They are empty of self. So is the Sage. He sits back in life, Yet finds himself in front. Dissolving his separation, He draws in Heaven and Earth, And pulses with the Cosmos, Achieving transcendent comprehension, The true aim of all Sages.

> *Dao De Jing* (Verse 7)

We have looked at how emptying the mind and energy system (and stomach) all have positive impacts on our level of physical and spiritual well-being. The question arises of how we can live in a world where our energy bodies and minds are bathing in the almost continual toxic presence of electromagnetic interference and emotional-sensory stimulation. Obviously, there is a balance to be had, as we neither want the reclusive life of a hermit nor should we succumb to the mind-numbing sensory saturation that our society encourages. It would signify a major failing of our internal development if we interacted with the world by recoiling from or indulging in it. The founding tenets of Buddhism clearly reinforce this point in saying that suffering at its root is caused by attachment and aversion.

The *Dao De Jing* (Verse 5) demonstrates the importance of equanimity as follows: 'The Sage is...without bias, Free of preference. Like and dislike have no importance, There is only what needs doing.'

It is important to remember that the philosophical and alchemical schools of Daoism existed long before the religious Daoist sects came into being. Daoism is not a monastic order that requires you to be divorced from the concerns of everyday life. Retreats are encouraged to catalyse certain processes in your training, but these are always alternated with periods of mixing with society. This is crucial because those characteristics that are born from stillness can be challenged and tempered by exercising them in worldly life. Such is the Dao of cultivating the Heart-Mind. When you attain a virtuous state of being it should not be shielded from exterior influences in bleak isolation; instead it needs to be strengthened until it reaches such solidity that even when exposed to the myriad forms that the chaotic nature of reality throws at you, it remains unbroken.

This benefits the people you interact with in addition to aiding your own higher-level alchemical practices. When your nature is rooted in stillness, the quality of your interactions with people becomes transformative. Rather than expressing and reinforcing the layers of your acquired nature, you begin to dissolve them in others to gently and passively undo the distortions accrued during their lives.

Less intuitively, this skill of acting from stillness is an essential trait used in internal alchemy. There is a stage in meditation (which I am nowhere near) where you begin to perceive various lights that signify that you have accessed the various alchemical ingredients. You perceive these through the 'window' of pure emptiness. In order to harvest these ingredients and draw them from the realm of emptiness into the realm of your body you have to reach through and 'grasp' them. However, in doing so you must maintain absolute mental stillness, otherwise the emptiness through which you are reaching is disrupted and disappears, along with your precious ingredients! This is a major reason why studying martial arts is so important in Daoist training. If you can remain calm and internally still whilst in the midst of mortal combat, then this ability is transferred into the sphere of meditation and facilitates more rapid awakening.

Unfortunately, we cannot survive in these meditative states for more than short periods at a time. By continually fasting mind and body you would starve and your body would waste away. As we can see through our practices, there are various points at which withholding stimulation to the mind and body produces enormous benefit. The lesson to be learnt is that, whilst beneficial, these states are not practical to maintain throughout the course of your life. They therefore become a clue as to how we should try to actively reflect in our lives the stillness that is the blueprint of creation that exists prior to the birth of the myriad things.

28

THE FIVE SPIRITS
OF DAOISM
Roni Edlund

The five spirits are a model of the different aspects of a person's consciousness and a major aspect of Daoist study. As well as this, the spirits help to govern various energetic and physical components of our internal environment. The individual functions of the five spirits are explained in Table 28.1 in relation to various aspects of the physical body system. Each of the five spirits are anchored into one of the five Zang organs because this is where the substances that form the material basis of the mind are produced and stored. These materials are Jing, Qi and Blood. In this way we can see that the Daoist view of life is to integrate the movement of human mind with the physical body as well as the movement of internal energy.

Table 28.1: The Five Spirits

Organ	Spirit	Material involvement
Heart	Shen	Invigorates the Blood with spirit
Spleen	Yi	Involved in production of Blood as well as the division and redistribution of fluids throughout the body
Lungs	Po	Helps to produce and invigorate Qi within the chest region of the body after absorbing environmental energy through the breath
Kidneys	Zhi	Combines the spirit of Yin and Yang with the rest of the body's energetic substances
Liver	Hun	Calms and stores the Blood

What follows now is a discussion of the five spirits of Daoism as individual entities. This discussion is based around a dissection of the Chinese characters for these spirits.

THE HUN (魂) THE ETHEREAL SOUL

The Chinese character for Hun comprises the radicals for Yun (雲) (cloud) and Gui (鬼) (ghost), as shown in Figure 28.1.

FIGURE 28.1: THE CHARACTER FOR HUN

Yun means clouds and signifies the Hun's ability to come and go as it likes, as well as alluding to its ethereal nature. The term 'cloud' also shows the ability of the Hun to rise to Heaven. The clouds are formed from the water of the physical world, and in the same way the Hun is dependent upon the denser spirit of the Po for life within the realm of manifestation. Clouds are associated with wind and pertain to the element of Wood, which is the element of the Hun. The second radical, Gui, means spirit or ghost – the top of the character shows a person's face, whilst the bottom of the character shows the disembodied nature of a ghost's form. Together this shows the ethereal – Yang – nature of the Hun spirit as well as its connection to the afterlife and the spirit world.

THE SHEN (神) SPIRIT

The character for Shen also comprises two radicals – Shih (示) (the sun, moon and stars and an altar) and Shen (申) (expansion of power). These two radicals are shown coming together to form Shen in Figure 28.2.

FIGURE 28.2: THE CHARACTER FOR SHEN

The first character is Shih; this radical depicts the sun, moon and stars and an altar. This is alluding to the Heavenly connection that extends into us through the spirit of the Shen. According to Daoist thought it was through these Heavenly bodies that a person could experience divine insight or inspiration. The second character, Shen, stands for an extension or expansion of power, showing how the spirit of the Shen can move through a person if they are able to contact it. Another interesting interpretation of this character is of a lightning bolt. Together this gives two different ways in which a person may be touched by their Shen – through expansion and divine connection or through the sudden shock of spiritual realisation.

THE YI (意) THE INTENTION

The first part of the character Yi shows a musical note. This denotes something that is being expressed externally into the world. Beneath this is the character for Heart, Xin (心). Here is a clear sign that the Yi and the Shen work closely together, since it is the Shen that is anchored into the physical root of the heart organ. Figure 28.3 shows the character for Yi.

FIGURE 28.3: THE CHARACTER FOR YI

Within esoteric and religious Daoist teachings it is the Yi that enables a person to utter chants, devotions and prayers to the Heavens, as these tributes to divinity rely upon the human intellect to be generated. It is also the Yi that receives the messages of Heaven via the Shen and interprets these messages into cognitive processes.

THE ZHI (志) OUR WILLPOWER

The top part of the character for Zhi shows a plant forcing its way up through the ground. This is clear representation of the necessity of Zhi for carrying out difficult tasks. Below this radical is, once again, the character for Heart. This is shown in Figure 28.4.

FIGURE 28.4: THE CHARACTER FOR ZHI

The character for Heart appears within both the characters for Zhi and Yi, as these aspects of mind have a dependency upon the Shen for their existence. The Zhi is the manner in which the Shen is rooted into the more Yin aspects of consciousness, whilst the Yi is the centralised interpreter of the Shen. This is in direct contrast to the spirits of the Hun and the Po, which do not contain the character for Heart. Instead these two spirits have a certain degree of autonomy from the rest of the human consciousness model.

THE PO (魄) THE CORPOREAL SOUL

The character for Po is made up of Bai (白), which means 'white', and Gui (鬼), which means 'spirit' or 'ghost'. The character for Po is shown in Figure 28.5.

FIGURE 28.5: THE CHARACTER FOR PO

In the case of the Po, the colour white indicates death and its connection to this aspect of the human soul. The Po is a mournful spirit, which will return to the earth upon our demise like so much spiritual compost. It is said that the Po, more than any other aspect of human spirit, is acutely aware of the nature of transience. It is this part of our spirit that is fully activated within human life at the age when we first learn that all human beings die. The second character of Gui or 'ghost' underlines the Po's connection to death. The Po works in partnership with the Hun to form the human soul.

Each of the five spirits are assigned various facets of human consciousness, and these are summarised in Table 28.2.

Table 28.2: The Mental Actions of the Five Spirits

Spirit	Activity
Shen	Receives insights and inspiration from Heaven
Hun	Planning, aspirations, dreaming, psychic gifts, ethics
Yi	Focus, awareness, short-term memory, expression, thinking
Zhi	Willpower, drive, clarity, long-term memory
Po	Sensation, feelings, instinct, mental stamina

Within Chinese medical theory it is the imbalance of the five spirits that is the result of psychological and emotional disturbances. Understanding the way in which these imbalances manifest can help us to understand not only the nature of the spirits but also why our mind works in the way it does. These imbalances are summarised in Table 28.3.

Table 28.3: Imbalances of the Five Spirits

Spirits	Imbalances
Shen	Mania, lack of inspiration, scattered spirit, insomnia, hysteria, sadness, depression
Hun	Delusions, hallucinating, psychosis, nightmares, sleep walking and talking, anger, frustration, jealousy, emotional swings, apathy, being overly judgemental, paranoia
Yi	Lack of concentration, poor focus, lack of expression, over-thinking, worrying, stuck thought processes, lack of sympathy, over-smothering behaviour
Zhi	Low willpower, lack of drive, no life goals, depression, being fearful, low self-esteem
Po	Emotionally numb, mind/body disconnect, lack of care for own well-being, over-indulgence, over-need for comfort, obsession with beauty, extreme vanity, sadness, grief, no ability to let go

When engaging in any Daoist practice, whether it be Chinese medicine or alchemical training, it is essentially these five spirits that we are seeking to regulate. If they can be brought to a harmonious state, they will become still and so a person will be able to move into higher states of consciousness.

29

TANTRIC DAOISM AND INTERNAL DEVELOPMENT

Linda Hallett

Key 'define Tantric Daoism' into your computer and all the information that appears on the first screen links Tantric Daoism with sex. A sad reflection on modern or perhaps Western society. The emphasis linking Tantra with sex rather than spiritual development perhaps shows how physicality takes precedence over spirituality in our lives. Try a search on 'Tibetan Tantra' and the root of the word reveals the original spiritual definition. Taken from the Sanskrit words 'Tanofi' meaning extend/expand and 'Trayati' meaning liberation, Tantra is defined as a practice that expands and liberates the mind. Tantra also has religious connotations, being linked to Buddhist and Hindu practices; one definition is given as 'a divinely revealed body of teachings on the practice of worship of god'. However, Tantra is not a religion but perhaps more accurately a spiritual practice. The aim is for the individual to gain an awareness/understanding that brings about a change in how they think and perceive themselves and the world. Sometimes referred to as an 'awakening', the individual begins to release their attachments to material things and shed their desires. As these changes occur the energy of the individual begins to unite with the energy of the universe, and they become content within themselves and thus attain spiritual enlightenment.

Try a search on Esoteric Daoism and links appear to mysticism, magic and alchemy. You are led down a path where there are possibilities of developing supernatural powers; you can buy magical mirrors and become clairvoyant! There are now Western schools where you can learn ancient Chinese magic and progress through the 'gradings' to become what? A magician? This is how the West is now marketing these ancient teachings. Is this really what these Daoist teachings are about?! I think not.

Esoteric means confidential information or teachings that are intended to be understood only by initiates within a group. Eva Wong in her book *Nourishing the Essence of Life* categorises Daoist teachings as shown in Table 29.1.

Table 29.1: Three Categories of Daoist Teachings

Outer teachings	Suitable for the public and novice practitioners Easy to understand Can be practised without teacher supervision
Inner teachings	Suitable for practitioners with a strong spiritual foundation Teachings more esoteric Texts and formal instruction from a teacher
Secret teachings	Most advanced esoteric teachings Only for the highest-level adepts Transmitted orally, direct from teacher to student

This shows the progression of training and spirituality required for a student to receive the inner Daoist teachings. Esoteric Daoism is the inner and secret Daoist teachings that have been carefully and selectively transmitted from teacher to student down through the millennia.

We may ask why the secrecy and why the connection to mystics, magicians and sexual practices. A brief history of Daoism explains these connections.

Daoism originated as the original philosophy of ancient Chinese people. It was based on following the Dao or the original way of nature, and many of the practices were aimed at returning to the source of life. The ancient people were attuned to the rhythms and energies of nature and their philosophy was to live in harmony with nature. Their shamans were said to have mystical powers of being able to commune with the spirits, interpret dreams, read omens, call on the heavens for rain and heal the sick. They were also skilled at celestial divination; by interpreting celestial changes the shamans were able to advise the imperial courts. These shamans were said to have magical skills of flying to the stars and travelling underground. They used talismans and incantations to heal the sick and ward off evil spirits.

This legacy has been preserved within certain sects of Daoism (Shang Qing (上清) Daoism), hence the references to magic and mysticism linked with Daoism today.

The references to sexual practices and Daoism stem from some internal alchemical practices. Some of these practices use the sexual act to cultivate the health and longevity of one practitioner at the expense of their partner. The practitioner must be totally free of sexual desire to gain the maximum benefit from the practice. If not free from desire the practices can actually be detrimental. Some Daoists consider these practices to be deviant and have labelled them the 'Crooked Path'.

Religious Daoism first appeared during the Western Han Dynasty (206–208 BCE) when the Han emperor dedicated a shrine to Laozi. It developed further with Zhang Dao-ling (張道陵) who claimed he had teachings revealed to him by Laozi. He became a religious cult leader, becoming a priest to mediate between the heavenly deities and the common people. The aim of many religious philosophies is to enable man to reach a higher understanding of his purpose and place in life. However, as with all religions, this was the turning point where a philosophy became manipulated by man for control and power over other people.

Although Daoist concerns about health and longevity are within the writings of Laozi's *Dao De Jing* and the Yellow Emperor's *Huang Di Nei Jing* (黄帝内经), this emphasis increased during the Warring States period (200–589 CE). Alchemical Daoism developed the arts for prolonging life and there was a strong belief in immortality. These Daoists worked on developing external and internal methods of cultivating the elixir of immortality. External methods included ingesting herbs and minerals and, from this, Chinese herbal medicines developed. Although the aim was a long life and immortality, many of these practitioners brought about an early death due to ingesting poisonous substances!

Internal alchemists worked with the internal vibrational energies within the body known as the 'San Bao' (三寶) or three treasures of 'Jing, Qi and Shen'. These three treasures may also be referred to as Essence, Energy and Spirit/Consciousness. They are ultimately the same energy that can vibrate at different frequencies, much the same as water can be transformed into ice or steam. The Jing vibrates just above the realm of the physical body and is refined through practice and converted into Qi. Qi is in the realm of the energy body and includes the meridian energy pathways, the etheric field around the physical body and the three energy centres in the head, chest and abdomen known as the three Dan Tien. The energy body channels energy to all the organs and tissues in the body. It can be felt through Qi Gong practice, as the practitioner learns to tune into their energy body, but is experienced by most individuals through the changes of their emotions. With further practices the Qi is refined to the higher frequency Shen or Spirit/Consciousness body, which can connect to the universal energy of Dao. Using various Qi Gong/Nei Gong techniques the ancient Daoist practitioners aimed to use these energies to cleanse the body, transform the mind and bring about a spiritual awakening and possibly immortality. It is these practices that strongly influence the modern-day esoteric Daoist practitioners. The aims remain the same as those of the ancient Daoists – long life, enlightenment and, for some really dedicated individuals, the possibility of immortality. To progress to the higher levels, Nei Dan meditation practices need to be developed alongside Nei Gong or internal skills. The practitioner will also require the guidance transmissions and inner teachings from a skilled teacher to progress to the higher levels of alchemy. These higher levels are still kept relatively secret, as some of the skills developed in training may be abused if the morality and ethics of the practitioner are not pure.

There are a number of reasons one may start Qi Gong/Nei Gong training. Practitioners may start training due to ill health and endeavour to improve their health through their practices. Some seek spiritual enlightenment and are initially drawn to the Nei Dan practices. Others may start within the martial arts and progress to the spiritual path. As the practitioner progresses, their aims may then change. The most seriously dedicated practitioners may still have the ultimate aim of returning to the source, connecting with the Dao and becoming an immortal.

Nei Gong works to transform the internal energies of Jing, Qi and Shen or 'San Bao'. These are the life-force energies of an individual. The aim in alchemy is to refine the denser Jing into Qi and ultimately to Shen. Shen is the most refined form of energy – the spirit or consciousness of an individual that enables them to connect with the universal energy of the Dao. There are a number of stages of Nei Gong that a practitioner must progress through to enable them to progress towards the ultimate connection with the Dao.

1. Conditioning the physical body.

2. Regulation of Breath and Mind.

3. Beginning Conversion of Jing to Qi.

4. Awakening the energy system.

5. Movement of Yang Qi.

6. Attainment of internal vibration.

7. Conversion of Qi to Shen.

8. Conversion of Shen to Dao.[1]

Where does the modern practitioner start their Nei Gong journey? Find a skilled teacher and look to the ancient Chinese classics for guidance. For example, consider conditioning the physical body. Following the Qi Gong practices of Da Mo's *Muscle/Tendon Changing Classic* or *Yi Jin Jing* (易筋经) is a good example of how these skills were used to strengthen the body. All Qi Gong practice should incorporate an initial stretching routine to open the energy channels and lengthen the tendons and the fascia. The Dao Yin Qi Gong sets are another example that helps to clear the energy pathways and stretch and strengthen the body. The Dragon Dao Yins are an excellent example of a Qi Gong set that can incorporate the physical stretches to strengthen the body and lengthen the tendons and fascia, whilst the energetic principles of breathing and focusing into the distance help to clear pathogenic Qi from the system.

Now consider regulation of the breath. Guidance is given in the *Dao De Jing*:

> *The sage knows when to seek progress and when to simply follow nature.*
> *Sometimes his breathing is forceful,*
> *Sometimes it is natural.*
> *Sometimes he creates expansion,*
> *Sometimes he simply succumbs.*

Dao De Jing (Verse 29)

---

1   Mitchell, D. (2011) *Daoist Nei Gong: The Philosophical Art of Change.* London: Singing Dragon, p.23.

The regulation of breathing is intrinsic to the practice of Qi Gong, Nei Gong and Nei Dan. Basic Qi Gong practices help the practitioner to learn to regulate their breathing. These skills are developed further as they progress with Nei Gong and alchemical meditative practices. When we are considering regulating the mind we may be aiming to focus the mind in order to lead the Qi or we may be aiming to silence the constant stream of mundane thoughts. The mind is described as the 'monkey mind' jumping about from one thought to the next. We are aiming to have a mind 'like a plough horse', just focused in one direction. The regulation of breath and mind act as communicators between the physical body, the energy body and our consciousness. Control of mind and breath is intrinsic to the progression of training. However, the control of breathing is easier to train than the control of the mind! If we are aiming towards enlightenment then part of the process is to settle the mind equally between 'the three bodies of man', i.e. the physical, energetic and consciousness within us. It is only when these 'three bodies' are healthy and functioning well that the mind can rest in the 'mysterious pass', which is the point of balance between all three.

Qi Gong exercises such as the Ji Ben Qi Gong may be used to start the conversion of Jing to Qi and for 'awakening' the Dan Tien. Again the *Dao De Jing* gives guidance:

He empties his heart mind,
Awakens his Dan Tien,
Rids himself of desires,
And strengthens his body.

Dao De Jing (Verse 3)

In Qi Gong practices we focus the breathing to quieten the thoughts that race through the mind. Focusing the mind and attempting to quell the 'desires' of the physical and emotional body is part of the process of balancing the internal energies. These desires may be for food, sex, money or power over others. These desires cause imbalances within the energy system, which then cause blockages or pathogenic energies to accumulate and hence illnesses to develop. Dao Yins may be used to clear these pathogens, whilst Wu Xing Qi Gong may then be used to nourish and strengthen the energies. We aim to balance the five elemental energies to quieten the emotions and so try to 'empty the Heart-Mind'. We 'awaken' the lower Dan Tien to activate the energy system by focusing our mind whilst breathing into the lower abdomen, guiding the Qi to the area. Once the lower Dan Tien is activated, the process of converting Jing to Qi and then Qi to Shen will start to take place. The movement of Yang Qi will happen naturally with continuous correct practices, and internal vibration will begin to develop. If the practices are maintained they can help the practitioner improve their health, shed their desires and attachments to the material world and gradually become a more enlightened being. Immortality requires further practice and access to an enlightened teacher!

30
TRANSCRIPT OF A CLASS
ON THE KIDNEYS
Part 1
Damo Mitchell

Within Daoism, the spine is sometimes referred to as the 'celestial pillar'. It is the aspect of the human body that runs like a horizontal column through our body, connecting us to the powers of Heaven above and Earth below.

Running through the centre of the human body is a long pathway of the meridian system known as the 'thrusting meridian' or 'Chong Mai'. This meridian branches out through the body in several different ways (Figure 30.1). One of these branches runs from the perineum to the crown of the head, while another branch runs through the centre of the spine. These are arguably the two most important branches of the Chong Mai.

According to Daoist cosmology, everything manifests on three different levels – physical, energetic and spiritual. This universal rule also applies to the thrusting meridian/celestial pillar – both at the level of Qi (meridian pathway) and the level of Jing (spinal column).

To the ancient Daoists, the health of the spine was vitally important. A healthy spine gives us a strong connection to the two powers of Heaven and Earth: it governs our relationship to the divine energy of pure Yang above and the condensed energy of Yin below. If the health of the spine is allowed to decline, our interaction with Heaven and Earth will become weak. Conversely, when our energetic and psychic connection to these two energies is insufficient, our spine begins to weaken and pain may be experienced. If the spaces between the vertebrae are allowed to close up, sickness will develop.

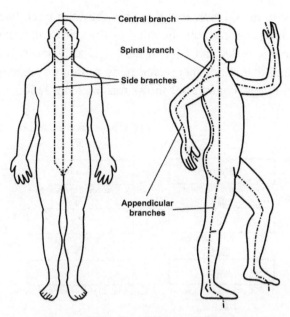

FIGURE 30.1: THE THRUSTING MERIDIAN

The Shen aspect of the celestial pillar is the element of our consciousness that runs through the centre of the thrusting meridian. It is a manifestation of the pure emptiness at the centre of our being that enables the force of Heaven to communicate with the five spirits. Thus, the celestial pillar acts as a 'spiritual antenna'.

Understanding imbalance, illness or spinal problems implies that we also look at the nature of disease according to the three categories of Jing, Qi and Shen (or physicality, energy and consciousness). Modern medicine works uniquely on the Jing layer. It treats sickness on the denser plane of matter and only addresses the body – in other words, that which is scientifically provable and measurable. Therapies such as Chinese medicine, acupuncture and Shiatsu aim to treat disease on the energetic level – the realm of Qi. Self-cultivation practices such as meditation and highly skilled energy therapists work on the level of Shen. Working directly with consciousness is a rare skill that is mastered by sage doctors.

Every disease or imbalance will manifest in the three realms of Jing, Qi and Shen. Disease cannot exist on one of these layers alone, as everything is reflected on all three planes. Here is a simple example. A physical injury affects the body – the realm of Jing. From there it will move into the Qi layer and then into the Shen layer. In the same way, something that disturbs the mind or the spirit will first manifest in the energetic realm and later in the physical realm. It is essential to understand that mind, energy and body cannot be separated – not until death, that is! Figure 30.2 shows this interconnection.

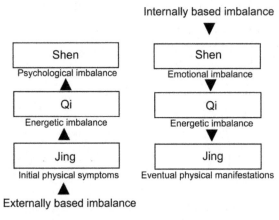

FIGURE 30.2: DISEASE ACROSS JING, QI AND SHEN

In mainstream modern medicine, a doctor will often treat a physical condition purely at the level of Jing. While this method will yield immediate results on the physical body, the energetic and consciousness imprints of the disease remain. This means that the condition will often return, either in the same form or in a different shape. Removing a tumour from the body may halt the progress of a degenerative disease in a very immediate kind of way; however, the root cause of this tumour is still there. This energetic information will continue to move through the body, causing imbalance. In time, the tumour may come back or another similar physical sickness may develop. Chinese medicine – or at least the way it is practised today – is also very limited, as it only treats the sickness on an energetic level. While rebalancing the Qi may help to ease the physical symptoms, the Shen layer remains untouched. The consciousness imprint of the sickness is still there and so the curative results will be temporary. This type of treatment is still limited. Few Chinese medicine practitioners have the skill that is required to treat the Shen; it takes many years of experience and a great deal of personal cultivation to be able to access the Shen. It is possible to shift someone's spirit through a Chinese medical treatment.

However, the responsibility for long-term spiritual change remains with the patient him or herself.

There is another obstacle that may prevent you from treating the spirit: even though you may have the skill to treat somebody's Shen, they may not be ready for this shift to take place. No disease can be completely cleared at the level of Shen unless the patient genuinely wants this to happen. Given a choice, hardly anybody would consciously choose to keep their spiritual ailments. However, the subconscious mind often thinks differently. Everything that we do or experience becomes a part of us and we end up having a 'vested interest' in many aspects of our being. This, sadly, can also include our ailments. Are we prepared to give up the part of our self that has grown around our illness? This can be especially difficult in the case of a chronic disease that has been with us for a very long time.

The process of the development and reflection of sickness across the three realms matches the Daoist theory of creation, as shown in Figure 30.3.

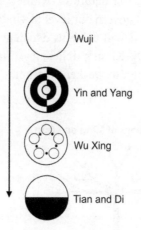

FIGURE 30.3: THE DAOIST PROCESS OF CREATION

Within the Daoist process of creation, Yin and Yang spring from the original void of Wuji, via the motive force of Taiji. The next stage is that of the five elements, which govern the transformational processes of life. Finally, the powers of Heaven and Earth come into existence. The process of creation can be seen as a gradual process of densification of an original vibration. As this vibration starts to change, the original 'nothingness' of Wuji gives way to physical matter. This process is reflected on a microcosmic scale in our bodies, when our emotions start to produce specific chemicals in the brain. Daoism would describe those chemicals as a physical substance (Jing) produced by the Shen. This is the process of consciousness transforming into matter. Between the two stages of Jing and Shen, there is also the manifestation of energy (Qi). The idea that consciousness produces reality is also matched at the level of the macrocosm; herein lie many of the principles of Daoism and indeed most Eastern spiritual traditions.

This process can be mapped out on an upside down tree, as shown in Figure 30.4. The development of sickness is represented through the trunk, branches and leaves, which respectively refer to the root cause, the sickness itself and the external symptoms. The roots represent the energies of Ming and Dao nourishing the tree. Let's now look at a specific imbalance from the perspective of Chinese medical thought. Kidney deficiency is the most common condition that Chinese medical practitioners will link to the health of the spine, so it would seem to be an appropriate example. Anybody who practises Chinese medicine will be familiar with the nature of Kidney deficiency. The Kidneys house the essence and govern our level of vitality. If our Kidney energy becomes depleted, this will make us deficient – which means we will start to run out of Qi. Kidney deficiency primarily affects the spine, knees and sex drive. It also weakens the immune system, as well as the health of the bones.

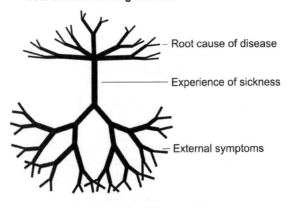

Nourishment of Ming and Dao

– Root cause of disease

– Experience of sickness

– External symptoms

FIGURE 30.4: THE TREE OF CREATION

Figure 30.5 shows the Kidneys and all their associated elements between the lower back and the coccyx. This curve in the lumbar spine contains the lower Dan Tien and the Kidneys themselves. A collateral branch of the Kidney meridian system runs from the lower spine into the Kidneys themselves and then the lower Dan Tien. This indicates there is a connection between these different aspects of the body. The three sections of the spine and the associated organs/elements of the energy body are divided into three sections. The lumbar section corresponds to Earth, the thoracic section to Man and the cervical section to Heaven.

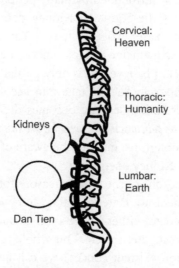

FIGURE 30.5: KIDNEYS AND THE SPINE

Kidney energy is closely related to the realms of Jing (physicality) and Earth. Depletion of this energy affects the physical structure of the spine and particularly the lumbar region, which is tied into the energy of Earth. Continuous depletion of this vital energy will begin to take its toll on the lower back. This weakness will also spread into the knees, attacking our very supporting structure – the Jing of our postural alignment.

Let's now look at the nature of Kidney deficiency from a consciousness perspective. The base desires are closely linked into the consciousness function of the Kidneys. The consciousness aspect of your Kidneys links you into the collectiveness or, on a simple level, your tribe/family or even society. Human beings are tribal creatures – pack animals. Most people now live in cities as part of an undistinguished mass of other people. We are not supposed to live like this. We are made to live in small groups; this is why human beings have an inbuilt desire to be a part of a unit. People who live on their own – completely isolated – normally become sick or eccentric. I have had the opportunity to spend time with many people living in isolation in Asia and I can bear witness to the fact that many of them were quite eccentric. Whilst isolation is good for periods of practice, it should also be remembered that our nature is to live as pack animals. Paradoxically, it is easy to become isolated when living in a city such as London, even when surrounded by many people.

So, what depletes the Kidneys? Kidney deficiency is a lack of vitality; it does not matter whether it is a Yin or Yang condition. According to Chinese medicine, we lose energy because of overwork, stress or excessive sex. I believe this is only partially true.

There is one important fact to take into account when trying to understand why our Kidney energy becomes depleted: *we are always choosing, consciously or subconsciously, why we are losing Kidney energy and in what form.* Even though we may not be aware of it, it is usually our choice to waste our Kidney energy.

In my experience, one of the biggest reasons for Kidney deficiency is people's attachment to material gains and wealth. Money is a curious thing that comes either in the form of small pieces of paper or as numbers in a computer system. Our whole economy and society are based on this non-existent concept we call money that only has strength because of the value people give to it. Of course, we all need money to live. Without money, we could not buy the things we need and pay our rent. Yet many people go beyond what is needed and endlessly chase the concept of money for the duration of their entire lives. This is fine, in theory. I guess it is what some people enjoy or they would not do it. Problems arise when we begin to attach our own energy to the money we are chasing.

Our Kidneys manifest the energy of our Zhi – our willpower – as well as how we view the will of Heaven as it passes through us. They also connect into that part of our nature that governs our sense of self. What is our will? What do we use to judge our own sense of self-worth? What do we link to our essence in an attempt to find some kind of gauge (with regards to how well we are doing and how well we are moving through life)? The answer to this depends entirely on us. We choose all of these things. It is our own acquired nature that decides for us what we are going to attach these concepts to, and I think that for many people this is money. How is this relevant? It means that all is good, as long as we are making money and we have enough. However, if we continue to chase this 'perceived wealth', we will end up losing our vitality as soon as we start to encounter any financial problems.

Let us look at other common objects that Kidney energy tends to attach to. A common one is attention and sympathy. Some people thrive off the attention you give them. They usually have some terrible woe in their life or an uncomfortable condition they are living with that makes their existence much worse than everybody else's on the planet. When you spend time talking to these people, you are left feeling drained – the very conversation is tiring. In alternative communities, these people are sometimes called 'energy vampires'. Once they have talked to you for some time about their problems, they tell you that they 'feel much better now, thank you', leaving you feeling exhausted. Why is this? Because their Kidneys got what they needed – they have attached their energy to sympathy and attention in the same way that others may attach their energy to money. Unfortunately, they have taken this energy from you.

At the opposite end of the scale, there are also people who derive their energy from their need to care for others. While this does not, on the surface, appear to be such a bad thing, it can cause problems when something bad happens to those that are being cared for. This disruption has a big impact upon the carer and so deficiency can arise. I was a social worker in the mental health field for a very brief period of time and I saw this many times with my colleagues. They were too energetically attached to their clients, and so when something went wrong or someone died it literally drained them. They eventually burnt out and ended up going off. The trick is to care without attaching, and I think this is a difficult thing to do.

A lot of people attach too much energy to relationships. In many personal relationships, one person is feeding off the other energetically and emotionally. This may sound harsh, but I believe it to be the case. If this applies to you, it is not such a big problem: you just need to ascertain why this is the case and then try to bring about some kind of balance. Some people *only* have energy if they are in a relationship. If that relationship ends, they quickly move on to another person so that the energy source is not taken away. These people are consumed with finding a new partner – nothing else matters until this happens. Sadly, this desire is like an empty heat, a fire fuelled on emptiness. Once back into a relationship, they become dissatisfied and so the energy source quickly fades.

This desire to find the perfect partner can also apply to other aspects of people's lives. This is the desire to find the perfect 'something' – the perfect partner, the perfect job, the perfect house or the perfect situation. All these things are noxious, as they cause the fluidity of the nature of Water to dry up. This lack of mental flexibility caused by a fixation on a single perfect point chokes the Kidneys, which lose their ability to keep flowing on the path of Ming. There is no perfect person, there is no perfect job, there is no perfect situation and there is no perfect purpose to life. There is just what is happening at this moment – this is all we need to understand. As soon as you define something, it becomes fixed. There is then no possibility for change or growth as the Kidneys become drained. A person's employment is a fascinating thing. Many people spend their whole lives working for large corporations, often in fairly low-level positions, and yet they still define themselves through this position. Perhaps someone was a janitor. While there is nothing wrong with being a janitor, it is wrong to judge your entire being through the role of being a janitor. Ultimately, most companies do not care about their employees. They care about making money to satisfy the Kidney essence of the person at the top of the pile; and yet, many of the workers make their employment the focal point of their very existence. What happens then? Well, they retire and die. The Kidneys were too attached to their role, and so once this is taken away they literally drop dead. Their existence has lost its purpose.

So, in conclusion, when trying to understand the nature of what is depleting our Kidney energy, I would suggest that it is wise to try and determine what we have created as a source of energy. This will necessarily be something transient, which means this energy is based on something very fragile.

Question from Student

When I am around people, I find that I become tired. Big groups really drain me and so I generally keep to myself and have little to do with people. Is this because people are draining me?

Damo's Answer

You should be careful of this. I know that you have practised Qi Gong for a long time now, and so it is important to become aware of how you fit into the rest of society. First, it is too simple to say that the people you meet are draining you. If you are losing your energy to groups of people, this is more likely an issue with how you attach to them. The problem could lie with how you see yourself in relation to them. I often hear internal arts practitioners state that they cannot mix with 'normal' people any more. They gradually become more and more reclusive until they are modern hermits, locked away in bedsits grumbling at all the 'unspiritual' people who are wasting their lives having pointless fun around them. It is common for a practitioner's 'dislike of people' to become a banner that they wave around. It becomes another layer to their acquired self that they use to elevate themselves above the masses. This is a trap that we must avoid. While short periods of reclusion are good for our practice, we must continue to live amongst other people and enjoy their company or it will only lead to loneliness. I am always a little disbelieving of many of the people I meet who live in virtual isolation all the time who say that they are not lonely. When I come across these people, they always seem incredibly pleased to have company. It is actually quite difficult to leave them, as they almost hold on to you for dear life when you want to carry on with your day! If you cannot be around people and you cannot stand to live as part of society, you must ask yourself what it is about you that is making these things difficult.

31

TRANSCRIPT OF A CLASS ON THE KIDNEYS
Part 2
Damo Mitchell

As with most spiritual traditions, a moment of conscious elevation is often accompanied by a bright white light. This light is a pure manifestation of the amalgamated spiritual elements that make up the Shen. When the five elements of human consciousness come together, even for an instant, this bright white light is manifested. This is the result of a direct experience of Yuan Shen (元神), our original consciousness. It makes me laugh when I think back to the stages of alchemy practice when I was in my early to mid-20s. I would experience this white light in my mind's eye while sitting. It would stay there, in front of my eyes, and then gradually begin to engulf my vision. After a while, it would feel as if I was looking into a pale sun. I had the strange idea that this light could only manifest internally; I had no concept that Yuan Shen could appear in the macrocosm of my immediate environment.

This all changed when I would repeatedly experience, over a period of several months, the white light of Yuan Shen suddenly coming down from above me and striking me at the top of my head or on the ground right next to me. It normally came with a feeling of warmth if it entered my body, and I became used to being hit by this light every couple of weeks. I was usually on my own, so I believed that this light could only manifest within the confines of my own mind (although it appeared to be outside my body).

One afternoon, the light struck me when I was not alone, for the first time. This occurred in my apartment in Cardiff (UK) when my student Neil was around. The light came down as before and I paid no attention to it. I then saw the look of surprise on Neil's face; he had seen the light as well. This happened again on a public course I was teaching in the UK when several of my students saw this light flash down into my head during a Qi Gong teaching event. The same thing happened while I was on holiday in Switzerland; this time, I was having dinner in a busy restaurant when the light hit me. I was sitting on my chair, feeling rather embarrassed and trying to pretend nothing had happened while the guests in the room looked bemused. I am not quite sure what that light was all about. The only thing I can think of is that I was going through emotional difficulties during that period – I wonder if this was related. Those strange lightning bolts have now almost completely stopped.

The point above me where the light manifested is known as the Kunlun point, which sits at the top of the etheric body, as shown in Figure 31.1.

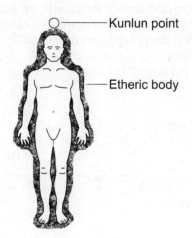

FIGURE 31.1: THE KUNLUN POINT

The point was named after the spiritual mountains on the northern border of Tibet. Meditation practitioners in both China and Tibet have used these mountains for spiritual retreats. Kunlun is the point of the eighth Chakra (Sanskrit term) in Daoism. In my experience, the light enters the auric body through the Kunlun point before dividing into five parts. This is perhaps easier to understand if you think of what happens when a white light passes through a prism – think of the cover of Pink Floyd's album *The Dark Side of the Moon*. After dividing into five parts, the light travels to five points on top of the head that mirror the five elements. The pathway of these lights forms a pyramid; this is shown in Figure 31.2.

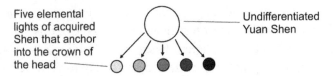

Figure 31.2: The Yuan Shen Pyramid

Question from Student

Are these points related to the Bai Hui (百会) (Du20) point and are they listed in acupuncture textbooks?

Damo's Answer

Yes, there are four points around Bai Hui, which are called the Si Shen Cong points (四神聰) ('four upright spirits') – 1 cun in each compass direction. Together, these five points absorb the light of Yuan Shen as it enters the auric body. Each of these points has an elemental relationship, as shown in Figure 31.3.

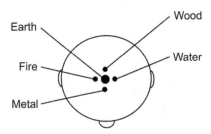

Figure 31.3: The Five Spiritual Points of the Crown

These lights then travel down into the body via the central branch of the thrusting meridian. They interact with the various key energy centres and other elements of our energetic system to produce the five base construct frequencies that form the five spirits, the five lights, the five tastes, the five movements and so on. This is the point from which Dao links into our energetic self. It is important to note that this connection is taking place at all times in each of us. However, we are able to strengthen this process through our practice; we can literally 'tune into' what is taking place at a higher degree.

It is through these energies, and through the central branch of the Chong Mai, that our mind interacts with our body. In other words, Dao interacts with our body via our mind and our energy system. The combined efforts of the five spirits, the Dan Tien and the three Jiao (三膲) (or burners) of the body enable everything to keep functioning smoothly.

Let us now return to our study of the nature of Kidney deficiency from a Shen perspective. We have already discussed how attachments can drain the energy of the Kidneys, but now let us look at the spiritual aspects of the Kidneys as they are associated with these five lights. The Kidneys are located in the lower Jiao of the body and they house the Zhi, which corresponds to our willpower.

The Zhi is our driving force. If the driving force of the Zhi starts to run dry, this causes the Kidneys to become drained, which will lead to weakness in the lower Jiao. The lower region of the spine is particularly susceptible to this type of weakness, as the internal branch of the Kidney meridian passes through the lumbar vertebrae. According to a recent study, about 70 per cent of Americans have some sort of back issue. It might be the case that Zhi weakness is a global issue. On the macrocosmic level, the Zhi directly ties into the will of Heaven, which is closely linked to our Ming – the nature of our path through life. How many of us are following the will of Heaven and how many of us are disconnected from that mandate with no sense of greater purpose?

So far, we have looked at the nature of Kidney deficiency according to its Shen aspect. Let us now look at how the body tries to rectify this situation. Daoism usually takes it for granted that the body will not deliberately do anything to hurt itself; on the contrary it will do what it can to make itself better. This means that if, for whatever reason, the Kidneys are drained, they will attempt to recuperate this energy in any way they can. Obviously, this sounds great; why not just let the body draw in the energy it needs from somewhere else? Unfortunately, it is the mind that selects where this new source of sustenance comes from. The mind is divided into two main parts: the acquired mind and the congenital mind. Our acquired mind is the conditioned aspect of our self, which can be likened to what many spiritual writers term 'the ego self'.

The acquired mind will generally try to draw in energy from wherever it can – even if, in the long run, it is not healthy to do so.

You may think of it as a kind of 'quick fix'. The energy sources that the Kidneys usually attach to will be based on something transient (as discussed above). For example, a person may develop an unhealthy attachment to status or an obsession with money or power, or they may want sympathy or attention. They are trying to draw in something to sustain the body's energy, although, in the long run, they will ultimately fail. On a personal level, we must be able to identify our own unhealthy attachments. As far as other people are concerned, it is not enough for us to understand their unhealthy attachments; we must also accept that they are the result of a deep suffering that drains their essence. Essentially, it is nobody's fault. Understanding is required to sever these attachments. Only then can we determine what can be done about a person's failing Zhi to repair the leakage of essence. This is the process of learning to stop 'propping yourself up' with flawed sources of vitality.

Question from Student

Does this theory apply to addictions then? Say alcohol abuse or drug use?

Damo's Answer

Yes, certainly. A person with a strong addiction has turned to an external source to try and fill the hole in their essence that has been created by something. This can be anything ranging from boredom and lack of purpose (poor Zhi) through to emotional pain. Addiction is closely related to the energy of the Kidneys and Zhi as well as the Po and Shen. Of course, as we know, these addictions ultimately lead to a person's health failing and often their death. Society is too quick to damn those with drug and alcohol addictions, though. The vast majority of people have an addiction of one sort or another; these addictions dictate every aspect of their behaviour and how they live their lives. This is always destructive and moves a person away from their true purpose in life. It only happens that drug and alcohol addictions are more visible and, as a result, have many stigmas attached to them. Is an attachment to money, power or even fast food any better?

It is interesting to me that these unhealthy attachments are key to many spiritual traditions' teachings. It is also at the point of some of these attachments beginning to change that the white light of the combined spiritual energies begins to appear. This is the stage of 'assimilating the material dust into brilliant light' discussed in esoteric Daoist traditions. You should recognise that these lights do not have to appear at a very high level in your practice; they can manifest in very early stages of training if you are able to recognise some of the attachments you have and allow them to begin to dissolve. Many of you will have experienced this, I believe.

I think it is much more difficult to end our attachments through an external approach, as opposed to the internal method I have just discussed.

Question from Student

What is the external method of ending attachment?

Damo's Answer

This would be a method whereby students are simply advised or instructed to end their attachments. They are given intellectual knowledge of what these attachments are doing and then a great deal of their focus becomes aimed towards ending all attachments or desires. In my opinion, this is an external method because it involves a teacher telling somebody what they must do. This is an intellectual method of ending attachment. It would be much like just listening to my advice and then going home to put it into practice; I do not believe it would really work. If I tell you right now to end all of your attachments, has it worked? Of course not. It would be the same if I told you to sit there and still your mind. These are very difficult things to do. Spiritual practitioners have struggled through history to achieve these goals. An internal method of ending attachment is based upon a practical method whereby the nature of a person's energy and consciousness are altered so that these attachments begin to fade. The ending of attachments is merely a by-product of what they are doing; this is the importance of ending all aims through training.

Let me give you an example. When I began looking into meditation in a serious way, I read all of the usual books people read. I had access to all of the usual teachings. I was surrounded by people who were amazed when their teacher told them to end all of their desires and attachments – in other words, their connection to the past and the future. Attachments are linked to our past, and desires are projected into our imagined future. These two things keep us from experiencing the very moment that we are living in right now. Now, all of this is wonderful in theory, but I could not really grasp the concept beyond this theoretical level. At the time, I was surrounded by many people who were greatly uplifted by this information. These people used to tell me with great certainty that they had ended all desires and attachments and now they were totally living in the present moment. I was very jealous, which obviously made things worse for me. It was not good for my Kidneys!

Over time, I stopped reading so many of these books and I continued with my sitting practice. I had become so despondent with my lack of progress compared with all the others who were now living 100 per cent in the moment that my personal aims for meditation practice ended; I had pretty much given up. Despite this, I continued to practise because it felt good and it helped me to relax. It was at this point of giving up that I really started to hit significant levels in my training. Allowing things to happen with no goal of ending desires and attachments continued for some time until one day I was having a conversation with a friend who I had known most of my life. The conversation turned to our past and growing up together. My friend discussed many things we had done – all the fun we had and some of the negative things that we had gone through together. He acknowledged that these events had shaped who he was and that our time together as children had been greatly influential in his life. Curiously, I found that I did not actually remember any of these events. I could not easily recall anything he talked about or indeed anything from this period of my life.

In fact, when I thought back to any time when I was younger I found that all my memories were hazy. I hardly remember my schooling, my teenage years or even up until my early 20s. I then discovered that if I try to project into the future, it is increasingly difficult for me to plan anything. I simply cannot see myself beyond the next year or so, no matter how hard I try. It is a definite feeling for me right now that my past and my future are closing in on me and the timeframe in which I live is restricted to only a few years; and this frame is growing smaller all the time. Rather than being worried about my ever-worsening memory, I actually see it as an aspect of the dissolving of my attachments and desires, my past and future.

As I continue my training, I continue to live ever increasingly in the present. This has the result of making me feel somewhat ageless; I have no past to judge my age on and so don't really have any concept of what point I am at on a lifetime scale. It is actually quite difficult for me to recall what age I am when people ask me. For me, this is an internal method of beginning to end all attachments and desires. It has brought me to the realisation that all of these ancient teachings on desires and attachments were not guidebooks as such – they were not telling you what to do, they were telling you what *you were going to experience through your training. This is quite a big difference.*

In summary, what is the use of living in the moment? What is the importance of ending our attachments and desires? Why do we wish to discover what our unhealthy addictions and connections are? In short, it is to help sustain the energy of the Kidneys and our essence. This will in turn help to sustain the power of our Zhi that helps us to move in line with the will of Heaven. When this virtuous circle is established, we can begin to connect to our sense of higher purpose and realise our full spiritual potential. This is the foundation of Daoism: the energy of water in action.

32

WHAT'S GOING ON?
Ellie Talbot

The day I found my way to Lotus Nei Gong, I sat on the floor looking around and asking myself, 'What am I doing here? This is mad!' Everyone was stretching, bending and twisting; it looked more like a Yoga or gymnastics class. At least I wasn't the only one looking bewildered. After a while we went upstairs to a small room for a short lecture to explain the principles of the Dao Yins. My legs were like jelly and wouldn't stop shaking the whole way through, while my head was having difficulty getting around these new concepts. I was used to doing what we sometimes refer to now as upright Taijiquan; this was something alien. The workshop I was attending was a present for my 60th birthday. The weather that day was foggy, miserable and gloomy. I had to take Peps the dog with me. She was so good, waiting outside in the car for most of the day. When it was time to leave, I was exhausted but exhilarated. I just knew that this was something I wanted to be doing for the rest of my life. That was the real beginning of a journey for me, and Peps and I would travel to classes and workshops together for the next five years.

I counted the years, the months, the days, the hours, probably even the minutes, until I could stop working. I always had physical jobs, moving and doing, because if I stopped I would just seize up. If I came home from work and sat down with a cup of tea, by the time I had finished it I couldn't move out of the chair again without a lot of effort and a great deal of pain. Joint pain, backache, tendon inflammation and muscle ache. I didn't just get tennis elbow, I had tennis thumb, tennis wrist, tennis shoulder and tennis collarbone. Even going for walks, supposedly 'gentle exercise' was out; it gave me tremendous lower back pain, so even Peps lost out. She would have to go for a 'mooch' instead of a proper walk. The muscle ache was in part due to the drugs I was given for angina. Not only did they cause the ache, but also each one lowered my blood pressure until I felt I could hardly function. The general response as to why my blood pressure needed lowering was 'just in case', so they all went out the window. I guessed I would probably be alright as long as I didn't overexert myself, and I had no ambition to run 100 yards, let alone a marathon. I bought various gadgets for opening bottles and cans etc. and some cycling gloves with gelbacks and wore them the opposite way round so that my palms had some protection when I put pressure on them to change gear in the car. I read a book on fibromyalgia and looked at the checklist of symptoms. I believe I ticked off about 19 out of the 20. That was it then; I became resigned to my fate because there was no suggested cure – medication yes, but no cure. I was already resigned in my mind to a downward spiral. You can easily find yourself falling into another weird kind of reality – one where people actually boast about their illnesses and the shedloads of pills they have to take every day. Fortunately for me, something else kicked in, which I didn't recognise at the time.

I saw a leaflet on the noticeboard in the local supermarket advertising 'Taijiquan classes' and felt an overwhelming urge to go. None of them fitted in with my work routine, but a few months later I changed jobs and when working out my hours, I requested one morning a week off so that I could go and see what these classes were about. I had never even seen anyone doing Taijiquan before, I knew nothing about it and it was weeks before I understood we were doing Qi Gong as well. Weird, different from anything I had ever done before, but fascinating, and I began to go week after week. At the end of each class I felt energised and developed my 'Tigger' legs. That's the only way I can describe it; as I walked up the hill towards home my legs had a discernible extra spring in them.

Since I began those classes, I have read many articles about Taijiquan, many of them in the general press usually recommending it as a gentle form of exercise for older people to help with their hips, knees and balance and to prevent them falling over so much, which would undoubtedly save quite a lot of money for the NHS. Not so much is written about the lowering of blood pressure, the destressing, etc. (Another complete chapter would be needed to mention the multitude of health and psychological benefits.) Although doctors seem to recommend it, I haven't come across any who actually practise Taijiquan and Qi Gong themselves yet (I would love to be wrong about this, but I have met quite a number of retired nurses). I have however come across many alternative medicine practitioners of all ages (I often find myself training alongside young, enthusiastic men and women in their early 20s). Could it be that they have a greater insight? Could it be that they have other skills – are they working with something else (energy work)? Something being a little difficult to explain or hard to understand at times doesn't mean that it doesn't exist.

When you don't know what you are doing, you copy. You trust your teacher (once you have found the right one), you listen, you watch and you mirror the movements. You become childlike again. I rarely take notes – not because I can remember everything, but because I seem to learn in a different way. The words or the principle behind them have to resonate with me before I can understand fully. I may have to hear or see something several times and make lots of comparisons, but that's okay – I've got time, plenty of time, all the time in the universe. I call it learning by osmosis.

For example, I have been taught that there are three basic types of Qi Gong: regulating, tonifying and purging. At the moment these are just words on a page. I have heard them often enough, I have repeated them myself and I have gone through the motions of the exercises many times. I have connected movements to meridians, organs, muscles, tendon collaterals, fascia and all the soft tissues. I have watched demonstrations and listened to lectures. I have watched people studying hard for years and making huge sacrifices to achieve their Qi Gong certificates. I have even taught some Qi Gong classes myself. But did I fully understand it? I don't think so. Why? Because it's not a thinking process – it's a doing-and-experiencing process. My brain is still partly in the 'hang on a minute' stage, while my body seems to have its own way of understanding. Could this possibly be the point where I'm beginning to be led into Nei Gong?

When we all meet at the courses and workshops I can't help but notice the changes (I tend to people-watch a lot of the time). Not just the smiling faces, there are so many subtle changes – the tone of their voices, the difference in the way they move, their energy and vitality, their body shape, the texture of their skin, a sparkle in their eyes, a radiance that sometimes stops me short and I have to do a double take. Many have improved with their practices; some have become teachers; some have even gone from 'Wimpy Kid' to 'Martial Artist'. Many have made life-changing decisions about their work, their studies, their lifestyles and sometimes their relationships. They talk about their latest exploits, experiences, travels and plans with a seeming lack of worry about what the future may hold. They are as they are supposed to be: 'on their own path'. They are blossoming.

What has happened to me? I don't keep a diary but I have a rough idea of what has changed. Timescales would obviously vary from person to person. I know that it has taken a full year to be able to change from leg facing inwards to leg facing outwards in the beginning warmups at my regular classes. My flexibility has improved, my muscles are stronger, I'm calmer and I'm a lot happier. Some changes have had to be conscious efforts and worked on; others seem to have appeared by themselves very slowly and subtly. The process has not been about going anticlockwise; I was never supple 20 or even 30 years ago and I have memories of bad cases of tennis elbow in my 20s. The chest pain I felt when doing school athletics – I thought was normal. While the regulating, tonifying and purging have been doing their work, the aches and pains seem to have shifted from one area to another and sometimes back again. I figured that I would never be free of it because, let's face it, until you can do a full stretch like the splits there's always a bit further to go (this is just my way of thinking; obviously we should all have a rough idea of our limitations). 'Pain is good,' says Damo with a grin, and usually adds: 'Just five more minutes.' 'Yeah, right' – I always thought it was meant as a joke. Pain captures our attention, disrupts our behaviour and motivates us to ensure our safety and end our suffering; I recently read that in a book about the brain (a light-bulb moment). To me, that means those of us who feel we're getting on a bit, and are feeling 'the oohs, the arghs and the ouches', don't just think it's the ageing process and that you have to grit your teeth and put up with it or with anything else that is making life uncomfortable; recognise it, focus on it, work with it and then release it. The pain shows the way (not just physical pain). Perhaps this is my brain finally catching up so that now I can begin to make the connections mentally as well.

My revelation began when Roni turned to me and asked how I had found the day's training. 'Yes,' I said, 'it was good.' 'Any aches?' asked Roni (I'd heard a few others mentioning where they felt stiff and sore). 'No,' I had said, but that I had felt one or two little clicks where I thought the bones were starting to shift into line a bit more – quite a peculiar feeling, almost as if they were reattaching in a different way.

'That's good,' she said. 'Perhaps you should write something about it to give some additional encouragement for older people who might like to come and train with us.' Even then I didn't twig. This was Sunday night when 22 of us were having a lovely meal in a Thai restaurant towards the end of the third day of the Zhan Zhuang (the standing post posture) course.

We arrived late at the hotel on Friday night after a long drive from North Wales to Bristol and began training at 9.30 the following morning after catching up with all our wonderful friends who had come from all over the world, along with a few 'newbies'. We trained until 5 pm, returned to the hotel, a quick change and then out on the town for a meal and a chat until late, then back to the hotel, more chat and then bed. This was repeated again on days two and three, starting at 9 am. Day four started at 8 am and finished at 4 pm. We said our farewells to everyone and were driven back to North Wales. We changed vehicles and went back to our own homes. I did a quick change and drove on up to my daughter's house up in the mountains and had a meal and a chat; it was 11 pm by then. 'So what have you been up to this time?' my daughter's family asked. 'Well,' I said, 'I've been standing in this posture for four days' – I demonstrated Zhan Zhuang (they always look at me as if I'm nuts) – 'and we went out and had some lovely meals.' The conversation then changed to types of food and favourite restaurants. They said they were tired and were going off to bed, so I went on up as well. It wasn't until I was alone in the bedroom that I got that light-bulb moment again. 'No aches,' I had said to Roni, and now here I was, finally going to bed after nearly five days' non-stop on the go, 'NO ACHES!' After the OMGs and the sit on the edge of the bed in a dazed state had passed, I thought back to my old checklist: headaches – er, no; muscle ache – no; joint pain – no; and so on and so on. It was amazing.

So what is going on? I'm not going to overthink the processes I've been through; I feel as though I have at long last begun listening to my body, particularly during and since the Zhan Zhuang sessions. My energy body has started to introduce itself and I quite like it; perhaps this is the 'real me' – the proverbial one that we all seem to be searching for. Who knows? I don't. Where are my limitations now? No idea – they've gone out the window too.

As for my gel gloves, they've been back in use, not for the same reason I bought them though. I took them to the retreat centre in

Sweden this year where I spent two wonderful weeks training in various martial arts. They fit quite neatly the right way round this time, inside the boxing gloves – the 'one size that fits all' – and protect my knuckles a bit more so I can land a decent punch. And as for the risk of falling over… I've no fears there; if I do, it will probably be me falling over laughing.

Don't stop me now 'cause I'm having a good time, having a good time!

33

THE PRACTICE OF COMMITMENT

Kulsoom Shah

Autumn has arrived and, with its inward draw, I have the opportunity to reflect upon this year and my time as a student of Lotus Nei Gong. Along with the rest of the students on the American Qi Gong certificate, I recently completed the third training for this year and, during the nine-day Dragon Dao Yin course, I had the pleasure of an insightful conversation with Tino about my practice and some of my difficulties regarding creating enough time to practise. I am certain that I am not the first student in this school to encounter this challenge, so here I am writing a chapter to share some of my experiences and thoughts on this matter and a little bit of what I have learned.

As a beginning student, the desire and devotion to train is quite strong. This is good because this is the time to sow the seeds for a consistent practice. After completing the first course in February, I returned home excited and eager to continue my training. I diligently kept track of my training in a journal and often trained for between three and four hours. This was good. I was exceeding the minimum requirement for the course (two hours). Often, I would become so engrossed in the training that I would lose track of time and find myself rushing out the door to make it to class/work on time. Training became the focal point of my life and everything else began to seem like a burden. Some would say I had an addiction. I trained compulsively every day until something in my life needed dire attention because I had been ignoring it. In this case, it was school: I had to study for exams, and because I hadn't been studying consistently due to my obsession with training, I had a lot of catching up to do. So, I switched gears and focused on studying (other than being obsessed with training, I also have very little patience for making anything less than an A); this meant that I went from training 100 per cent and studying 0 per cent to training 0 per cent and studying 100 per cent. Clearly, the scales were tipped to the extreme in both cases. I finished the semester keeping my sanity and my GPA (grade point average), but training suffered for a few weeks.

Those of us who have a strong disposition towards the Metal element can relate to this. Balance is sometimes difficult to come by because the drive for perfection is the fuel behind every endeavour a Metal personality is committed to. I recognised this and realised that I had to create some balance in my life, so I created a timetable of all my daily activities and created a two-hour time slot for training at the same time every day. This lasted for a few days, because life is unpredictable and never goes as planned. At this point, I started training whenever time became available. My training got broken up into sections: stretching in the morning, strengthening around lunch time and Qi Gong/Dao Yin whenever there was a chunk of time available at home. I would do breathing practice in my car in between classes or go stretch in the Taijiquan room during breaks. I even started sitting at the back of the classroom so I could get up and stretch instead of remaining seated for the entire duration of a three-and-a-half-hour lecture. Although I wasn't training for as many hours as I wanted or with as much focus and consistency that I desired, I was still training, and that seemed to be the best I could do at the time.

After the most recent training my perception about training has shifted significantly. This came about in part due to my conversation with Tino and also because one of my peers at school asked why I was willing to miss nine days of classes and clinic to go to training. My colleague pointed out that the traditional Chinese medicine (TCM) programme we are a part of is too rigorous, so she doesn't have time for anything else in her life other than university. This is a sentiment echoed by several of my other colleagues as well. When I was reading Damo's book, *Heavenly Streams*, in the lunch room, I was asked how I had time to read anything other than textbooks. Such comments have made me realise that many of the students at my school fuel themselves with coffee and energy drinks, are often complaining of feeling exhausted and are waiting to complete their Master's degree so they can get on with their lives.

When I was first questioned about how I had time to read non-course-work-related books and take days off to go training, I felt guilty. I felt as if I was a bad student, a fraud, for not focusing my entire life on being a student. My entire undergraduate experience was spent mastering the student persona: study sessions that ran up to four in the morning followed by an espresso shot and then on to take an exam. I placed value on being the tired student with a cup of coffee in her hand. 'It's the student life,' I would often find myself saying. Sure, I graduated with honours but had nothing to show for that GPA other than poor health and depression. I became a student of TCM because I wanted a healthier lifestyle, and when I learned that the institution I am studying at is no different than any other educational institution, I jumped at the opportunity to study with Lotus Nei Gong.

Now, it's really easy to answer my colleagues when they ask me how I have time to train: it's because I value training. Clearly, the practice feels addictive because it's good for my body. Sure, sometimes the practice is very challenging physically and emotionally. Oftentimes, it feels as if my entire sense of self is defragmenting, but at the end of the day it's worth it because I know myself better now than I did last year. The noise in my head has subsided. A sense of peace and serenity pervades my being and most days I am able to observe my emotions displayed on a blank canvas instead of being caught up in their currents. All of this is good and I cannot imagine not training, because the days when I don't train I can feel my body tighten and my mind become chaotic – and that is not what I value.

Although I still don't have the perfect formula for creating a consistent training practice, a deep sense of gratitude fills me because I have the time and opportunity to train and integrate what we learn on courses into my daily life. It's apparent to me that, back in February, I did not know how to carry my training into my life and throughout my life. There was a clear distinction between time for practice and the rest of my life. Practice is life, or life is practice. Perhaps both are true.

'Just keep smiling.' Tino's words continuously echo in my head. These words are a constant reminder to me of how I can begin to carry the practice into the rest of my life. When the corners of my lips turn up, I feel my neck straighten and shoulders relax. My body has begun to recognise the triggers. Instead of feeling anxious about creating time to practise, now I know that my body knows the importance of practice, and the time to train will make itself available just as it has been.

In summary, I can offer three words that are a constant reminder for me when it comes to having a consistent practice: commitment, compassion and value.

- Commitment: Having a consistent daily practice is a matter of commitment and I make this commitment to myself every day – to train even if I don't have a huge chunk of time.

- Compassion: Being a Metal-element person, I can be hard on myself and I have learned to have compassion for myself and for this process. I don't beat myself up if I don't train for four hours, but when I do have four hours to train, I go for it.

- Value: It's a good practice for me to check in with what I value and always choose to commit to the things I value. I value my health and I value my practice, so I choose to commit to them every day.

So keep smiling and keep training!

34

KNEE PAIN IN THE
INTERNAL ARTS

Richard Agnew

Knee pain is quite common among practitioners of the internal arts and is something I have struggled with myself when doing extended periods of Zhan Zhuang or Qi Gong exercises that involve a lot of standing. Knee pain is usually experienced because of some incorrect alignment in your posture, though sometimes there are longer-term structural issues. In theory, these structural misalignments should resolve over a period of correct practice, but this may take some time and there may be specific exercises that can help. The purpose of this chapter is to highlight some common alignment mistakes that can result in knee pain, as well as talking briefly about some of the less common structural issues that can be involved.

The knee is designed to be a stable joint – the body weight should pass evenly through the knee joint to be transferred to the foot and the ground. If the knee joint is not stable and balanced, the force will accumulate in the knee, creating pressure on the joint. Figure 34.1 shows the correct alignments for standing practice.

- Keep your feet parallel.

- The legs should be bent into an arch shape.

- Make sure your knees don't extend beyond the toes.

- Keep your body weight over the Yong Quan (K1) point, behind the ball of the foot.

- Bend from the Kua, with the sacrum neither pushed backward nor tilted forward.

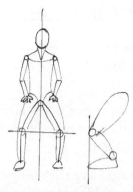

FIGURE 34.1: CORRECT ALIGNMENT (STANDING)

LIST OF COMMON ALIGNMENT MISTAKES

- Knees beyond toes: Usually more of an issue in lower stances, but make sure your knees do not extend forward beyond your toes. This will put pressure through the front of the knee.

- Feet not parallel: This creates a twist on the knee and tends to drop one or both knees inward, putting pressure through the medial (inner) side of the knee.

- Feet not level: This creates a twist on the pelvis and also tends to drop one or both knees inward, putting pressure through the medial side of the knee.

- Both knees collapsed inward: Most people have tightness in the Kua (or groin area) – the leg adductors. When they completely relax into a standing posture, this tightness will tend to pull the knees inward, again putting pressure through the medial side of the knee. Although relaxing the body is vitally important in Qi Gong, the muscles still need to be engaged sufficiently to maintain the correct structure.

- Weight too far forward over the ball of the foot or toes: Here the knees are not beyond the toes, but the body weight is distributed too far forward over the feet. This will not only fail to open the Yong Quan (K1) point, but may also put pressure through the front of the knee.

RESOLVING COMMON ALIGNMENT MISTAKES

- Use a grid: Stand on a floor with square tiles, wooden beams or painted lines to ensure your feet are lined up, level and parallel.

- Use a mirror: Check your knees aren't dropped inward by practising in front of a mirror (or video your practice if you are moving around lots).

- Stretch out the Kua: Since most people have a tight Kua, and this is not only useful for correcting postural errors but also for opening up these major energy gates, it is a good idea to stretch out the Kua at least once or twice daily.

Two Simple Stretches for the Kua

1. Each morning and evening, lie face up in bed with the soles of the feet touching and the knees bent out to the sides. Drape a heavy quilt or duvet over your knees to pull them gently downwards. This is shown in Figure 34.2.

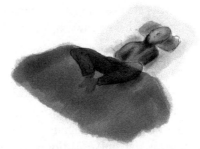

FIGURE 34.2: STRETCHING THE KUA

2. Lie face down on the floor, with the soles of the feet together and knees apart. Use your body weight to gradually stretch the Kua open and bring the body closer to the floor. This exercise is shown in Figure 34.3.

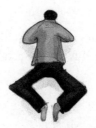

FIGURE 34.3: ALTERNATIVE STRETCH FOR THE KUA

OTHER STRUCTURAL ISSUES

Tight Iliotibial Band/Tensor Fasciae Latae

The iliotibial band (ITB) runs down the outside of the thigh, connecting the pelvis (via the tensor fasciae latae or TFL) to the shin bone. When this tightens up, it pulls on the lateral side of the knee.

RESOLVING TIGHT ITB/TFL

1. Lie on your side on a foam roller or tennis ball and slide along the foam/ball so it presses into the tight tissue on the side of the thigh. Slide up and down for a couple of minutes to release the tightness in the tissue. Repeat every day.

2. Get some cupping/massage/acupuncture/rolfing regularly, as these approaches may be able to draw out stagnation from deeper within the tissue.

Weakness of Vastus Medialis

The vastus medialis is the most medial (inner side) of the quadriceps (the thigh muscles). It is a key stabiliser of the knee and tends to become weak. This reduces the stability of the knee, which can exacerbate other small imbalances.

RESOLVING WEAK VASTUS MEDIALIS

Sit in a chair facing a wall, with one foot against the wall. Push forward with your toes for about five seconds. Rest for about five seconds, then repeat. Do ten repetitions with each leg twice a day.

Weak Gluteal Muscles

The gluteal (buttock) muscles are a key stabiliser of the hips and lower back. When they are weak, this causes instability that can in turn affect the knees.

RESOLVING WEAK GLUTEAL MUSCLES

1. Lie on your side with your knees bent at about 90 degrees and hips at about 45 degrees, then raise your upper knee, keeping the feet together. Hold this position for a few seconds, then bring the knees back together. Do ten repetitions with each leg twice a day. This is shown in Figure 34.4.

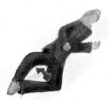

FIGURE 34.4: RESOLVING WEAK GLUTEAL MUSCLES

2. Lie on your side with your legs straight, then raise the upper leg to about 45 degrees. Do ten repetitions with each leg twice a day. This exercise is shown in Figure 34.5.

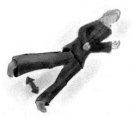

FIGURE 34.5: ALTERNATIVE METHOD FOR WEAK GLUTEAL MUSCLES

'Dropped' Arches

This refers to the arches on the medial (inner) side of your feet. Despite the name, they usually haven't dropped so much as never really developed in the first place. This changes the angle of the ankle, causing the knee to drop inwards, the pelvis (and Kua) to close and the piriformis (another muscle in the buttock) to tighten up.

Resolving 'Dropped' Arches

1. Squeeze your foot against the floor, aiming to bring the ball of the foot closer to the heel. Hold for a few seconds and do ten repetitions with each foot twice a day. Try not to scrunch up the toes.

2. Practise picking up a towel with your feet.

3. When standing (especially when practising Qi Gong or other internal arts), aim to put your foot into the correct position as in point 1. Remember not to scrunch up the toes and don't roll out onto the lateral (outer) side of the foot. You may need to engage the gluteal muscles to avoid creating a twist on the knee.

4. It is very difficult to build up arches if they haven't developed properly at a young age, so unless you're practising for many hours a day, the exercises above may not be enough to put you into the correct position. Orthotics are special insoles for your shoes that can help by putting the foot into the correct position. Orthotics won't help you build up your arch, but can alleviate many of the structural issues that happen further up the limb, including knee pain. You can buy off-the-shelf orthotics, which are probably okay for most people, or you can visit a podiatrist or other health professional who specialises in gait analysis for custom orthotics.

KNEE JOINT AND OTHER PROBLEMS

There are also quite a few problems of the knee itself such as arthritis or bursitis, and back issues causing sciatica can result in pain in the knee, but generally these issues will be more noticeable during daily life as well and not just while you're doing standing Qi Gong or similar exercises.

CONCLUSION

There are quite a few causes of knee pain, and this chapter has only touched on some of the most common. Look at the common alignment mistakes first, ask your teacher for help and, if you're at all uncertain, it's probably a good idea to get properly diagnosed by a professional. Physiotherapists, osteopaths or chiropractors are usually your best bet.

35

YANG SHENG FA

Part 1

Rob Aspell

Good health is not about never becoming unwell nor never getting injured – everyone gets injured or unwell at some point in his or her life. Good health is about how well your body can recover. A healthy body and mind will recover quickly and efficiently, injuries will repair smoothly and the mind (Shen) will be open and learn from the experience. Here I want to introduce the concept of Yang Sheng and discuss briefly how and why a practitioner should go about self-cultivation, and how it can improve their health and daily practice by giving the principles of Yang Sheng application for day-to-day life.

> It is man himself, not Heaven, who governs his life, and he who abuses himself dies young, while he who takes good care of himself enjoys a long life. (Gao Lian, Ming Dynasty)

Maintaining good health and well-being is almost uniquely characteristic to Chinese medicine and culture. Chinese medicine literature contains theories on both curative medicine and preventative medicine – Yang Sheng Fa is based on the latter. Translated roughly as 'life-nourishing principles', Yang Sheng Fa is the art of enabling self-cultivation by taking our health into our own hands and acting to prevent illness and preserve optimum well-being. It is a lesser known, but highly important, concept in Chinese medicine, and can be considered a philosophy of life. Yang Sheng Fa promotes methods of self-healing and health cultivation and encourages a positive state of mind, ultimately leading to the preservation of one's health, well-being and, from a practitioner's perspective, greater focus and training/treatment outcomes.

The art of Yang Sheng Fa is less about teachings and more about principles. Developed largely by the famous Daoist doctor Sun Simiao, little information about Yang Sheng appears to be available in the West, with even less actually referring to it as Yang Sheng. Small descriptions however are present in the Chinese medicine classics, such as the *Huang Di Nei Jing* (*Yellow Emperor's Inner Classic*), and authors such as Daniel Reid talk extensively about health preservation from a Chinese medicine perspective. There are many aspects of Chinese medicine, and Yang Sheng Fa lends itself to the branches that can be used by yourself without having to visit a Chinese medicine practitioner. These methods include:

- food therapy/dietary improvements

- herbal supplementation

- living with the laws of nature

- mind cultivation

- acupressure/self-massage (Tui Na (推拿) or An Mo)

- energy/breathing exercises (Qi Gong)

- physical exercise (Dao Yin or other movement exercises such as martial arts).

Yang Sheng can be a way of taking *advice and training* on health and well-being, and tailoring it to your own individual needs and preferences. It was believed in ancient times that a practitioner of Chinese medicine should adhere to what is known as Yang Sheng Fa in order to cultivate themselves as therapists. However, it is understandable that not every practitioner can strictly follow each component of Yang Sheng, though adhering to certain aspects of it can unquestionably help.

Recently in my own health clinic, a growing number of patients have been requesting treatments simply for health preservation and asking me to teach them about ways in which they can 'self-medicate' based on classical Chinese medicine. As a practitioner of Chinese medicine, this is exciting to me, as patients who adhere somewhat to the principles of Yang Sheng appear to react much more strongly to my therapy, much in the same way that acupuncture, Tui Na and Chinese herbal medicine support each other. It is simply adding another tool to the collection. For instance, if I am treating a patient to clear heat and enrich their Yin, yet that patient's diet largely consists of foods with hot and drying properties (Yang in nature), I will be fighting an uphill battle. The choices that I make in regards to herbal formulae, for example, need to be supplemented by Chinese food therapy. After all, both are being digested, transformed and transported in similar ways. Should I not offer advice on certain aspects of Yang Sheng, that patient will be undoing all the work for which they came to me in the first place, thus wasting both of our time. This is just one reason why it is important to give patients aftercare advice and explain to them what they need to do in order to cooperate with the treatment plan.

Ultimately, what is equally important, in my eyes, is how essential it is to understand the importance for a practitioner (whether in Nei Gong, Chinese medicine or something else) to implement at least some aspects of Yang Sheng Fa into their own daily life should they wish to offer optimum levels of treatment, get the most out of training and themselves remain in good health. From what I hear, too few practitioners, especially in the West, are aware of, let alone practise, any part of Yang Sheng. This and the following chapter will introduce you to the very basics of Yang Sheng and explain how it can benefit the practitioner, in addition to the patient. The study of Yang Sheng can be complex and covers many, many aspects of life. However, I do believe that a difference can be made to one's health and practice just by starting out with the basic understandings outlined within this and the following chapter, and it should, I hope, spark an interest and lead on to further study of the aspects that apply to and best suit yourselves.

CHINESE FOOD THERAPY

Our Yi is one of the five Shen and is the spirit that pertains to the Spleen; our Yi gives us our intent, focus and clarity of thought. Due to the fact that it is 'housed' within the Spleen and therefore affected by the well-being of our Spleen, the strength of our Yi is directly influenced by the quality of our diet and condition of our Ying Qi (nutritive Qi). If our diet were poor, our Spleen would struggle to function at its optimum, and our Yi can become unsettled – this is the point when our intent becomes unclear and our mind struggles to focus.

> Medicine is intention (Yi). Those who are proficient at using intention are good doctors. (Sun Simiao)

It could be argued that in order for a Chinese medicine practitioner to become a great practitioner, they must to some extent follow the principles of Yang Sheng. In the *Huang Di Nei Jing* (*Yellow Emperor's Inner Classic*), Qi Bo states: 'The key to acupuncture is first of all to concentrate and focus... When manipulating the needles with your fingertips...focus all of your attention.' On the one hand, this suggests that one must concentrate on inserting and manipulating in order to perform the correct technique, requiring a clear mind and focused thought. On the other hand, one could argue that Qi Bo is talking about focusing and transmitting one's intention, and therefore Qi, into the needles. This is mentioned in other Chinese medicine texts and is also suggested in the quote above by the great Daoist physician Sun Simiao. The ability to do this would be much stronger depending on the strength of the practitioner's Yi and shows that it is even more important for the practitioner to be healthy, as one should not transmit unhealthy Qi into a patient. Either way, it explains the importance of the practitioner having a clear mind and strong, healthy intent. Only through this can one take that extra step towards being a better practitioner. This is equally applicable to a Nei Gong practitioner. When training in practices such as Nei Gong or Dao Yin, it is very important to have strong Yi and to be able to identify or engage with our Yi. If the Yi is weak, a student or practitioner may begin to wrongly apply their Zhi (willpower) to lead and direct the Qi, which will ultimately weaken the Kidneys and pre-natal Jing and therefore cause further detriment to their health. A healthy diet is the first step to being able to engage our Yi.

Food is fuel – would you put low-quality fuel, or even the wrong type of fuel, into your car and expect it to run smoothly? The food that we eat has a direct influence on our Qi. Our Spleen is 'the sea of Qi and Blood' and is also the source of our acquired Qi. It is what gives us our energy to function. Without proper nourishment through diet, our Ying Qi and Wei Qi levels would become low. This will lead to fatigue, dysfunction of the Zang Fu (脏腑) and low immunity to disease. As practitioners, we need our Qi to be strong and healthy, and our Zang Fu to be working in harmony, in order to treat or train day by day.

'Food should not be eaten too hot or too cold.' This statement refers to both the temperature and property of food. Extreme temperatures, such as ones that burn the mouth or ones that are too cold for the teeth, cause the Stomach and Spleen Qi to weaken respectively. This is due to the fact that the Spleen and Stomach's function of transforming and transporting requires the food that you have ingested to be of body temperature, so that it can easily be absorbed and digested. Too cold, and the Spleen's functions will have to work harder, thus damaging the Yang Qi of the Spleen. This is reflected in studies of modern medicine, where it is said that for the alimentary canal to proficiently absorb nutrients, the food substances are required to be at body temperature. If food is too hot, the Stomach (a naturally Yang organ, which therefore likes colder substances) will become Yin deficient, which may give rise to Stomach Fire and damage to the Yin fluids.

The nature of food, which in Chinese food therapy (and herbal medicine) are Hot, Warm, Neutral, Cool and Cold based on Yin and Yang theory, can relate to the Yin and Yang of the organs. Therefore, the properties of food can alter the body's balance of Yin and Yang, depending on which channels and organs the foods enter from a Chinese medicine perspective. For instance, a patient suffering from Heat in the lungs with dry cough should stay away from black pepper, as this enters the lungs, dries phlegm and warms the body. Black pepper would thus be too warming and drying for that specific patient. By following food therapy from a Chinese medicine perspective, one can eat foods based on syndrome differentiation and cook meals according to their current condition. Should one follow these principles, food alone could arguably treat disease or in the very least aid the function of Chinese herbal medicine or acupuncture by acting as an agonist, rather than an antagonist. Simply advising patients to eat or keep away from certain foods could vastly improve the efficacy of the treatment. Likewise, eating or avoiding certain foods based on current imbalances during Nei Gong practice can improve progression. There are many books now available that contain tables and lists of different foods and their properties, and reference to these can be invaluable in treating some stubborn diseases in addition to health management.

Having meat is important, as is having vegetables. Some diets may suggest cutting out meat altogether, whereas other diets focus on meat being the main substance. There is a large amount of disagreement in the West in regards to the inclusion of meat in one's diet and whether or not its positive effects outweigh the negative ones. Meat contains many nutrients that the human body needs, and in the autumn and winter seasons can warm the body and prevent the intrusion of cold. Too much meat however can cause a build up of phlegm and cause too much heat within the body. This is reflected in modern research, which has found that a meat-rich diet can increase the risk of certain cancers.

In respect to the Yi, meat can stiffen the mind and cause difficulty focusing. To prevent this, the inclusion of vegetables alongside meat is a necessity. Vegetables promote digestion and can clear the intestines and stomach of phlegm and stagnation. However, although vegetables do contain many needed nutrients, vegetables alone do not provide the body with all that it needs – therefore a comfortable mix of both vegetables and meat (with vegetables being the main focus) is a must for a balanced diet. Daoist thought is that everything in life should be taken in moderation – even moderation!

In regards to moderate eating habits, too much food can damage the Stomach and Spleen due to overconsumption, whereas too little food will cause the body to lack nutrients. Both will likely lead to ageing of the body. Bigger meals should be eaten in the morning, when the Qi of the Stomach and Spleen is at its strongest and most active, and little should be eaten in the evening in order to prevent a build up of food stagnation and damage to the Spleen Qi whilst sleeping and disturbing the Heart and Shen. Most have heard the saying 'Eat breakfast like a King, lunch like a Prince and dine like a Pauper'. This seems to go against what is the 'norm' in modern society, and may be difficult fitting around today's busier schedules, but it is hugely beneficial if it is done.

Chinese food therapy is a vast subject in its own right, including how things are cooked, when they are cooked and with what – combinations of foods. Justice cannot be given to this topic in just this short introduction. These are the very basic principles. Food can be prescribed and consumed as medicine. It is the original and the best medicine. There are countless books on the subject, and you should look at the guidance they offer.

DAO YIN EXERCISES

Like other aspects of Chinese medicine, Dao Yin exercises are based on the ancient theories of Yin and Yang, the Wu Xing (five phases) and the Qi circulation throughout the Jing Luo, specifically the Jing Jin (tendon collaterals). The body is again seen as a whole – thus the fundamental concept of holism in Chinese medicine also applies to Dao Yin.

> Ageing does not occur with bodily movement. (*Lu Shi Chun Qiu* (*Lu's Spring and Autumn Annals*))

Dao Yin, literally meaning to guide and to stretch, are sets of exercises that are generally more Yang in nature than Qi Gong (energy/breathing exercises) and were developed for the practitioner to stretch along the Jing Jin, to guide the Qi and Blood in order to prevent stagnation within the Jing Luo and to balance the Yin nature of Qi Gong and meditation. They were designed to help the practitioner release tensions from within the muscles and tendons and to promote the Qi, Blood and body fluids to flow in and out of the joints and the Qi Men (Qi gates), flushing out toxins along the way. They are said to be important in purging the negative pathogenic factors from within the body and extending the mind to allow them to exit the body.

The importance of regular exercise and its beneficial effects on health and lifestyle is becoming increasingly apparent. For this reason Dao Yin exercises are a particularly useful daily practice, for self-use as a practitioner and for patient aftercare advice. Tui Na (Chinese medical massage) for instance can be a rigorous workout for the practitioner. If one's body is not prepared, it can be a matter of just a few treatments before the practitioner's Qi becomes deficient and stagnates within the muscles and joints. This can be quite detrimental over a long-term period – such as that of a Chinese medicine practitioner's career. Much like with the aims of a Tui Na treatment, there needs to be a fine balance between strength and relaxation of the muscles, tendons and sinews for the body's physical structure to remain healthy. Physical exercises such as Dao Yin exercises can help prepare and stretch the practitioner's muscles and joints, and combined with Qi Gong will help the practitioner to retain healthy, free-flowing Qi. Furthermore, movements within Dao Yin exercises are smooth and low impact, and can be done by almost anybody in only a few minutes if time is restricted.

The specifics of Dao Yin exercises are too great to go into within this short chapter, though there are again some great books on the subject. There are many types of Dao Yin exercises that have been developed over the past few thousand years, some of which were the basis of creation of the Wu Qin Xi (Five Animal Frolics) by the esteemed Daoist physician Hua Tuo, who adopted the principle: 'Ageing does not occur with bodily movement.' Other famous Dao Yin exercises are those of the Ba Duan Jin (Eight Pieces of Brocade) described by Sun Simiao in the book *She Yang Zheng Zhong Fang* (*Handy Prescriptions for Health Preservation*).

36

YANG SHENG FA
Part 2
Rob Aspell

A lthough mental nourishment is not as specific as the physical nourishment of food therapy, nor does it have a specific corporeal form like Dao Yin, its importance to the preservation of one's overall health should not be overlooked, as it so often is. Over the centuries, many different cultures have come to the conclusion that spiritual cultivation plays a large part in health preservation and longevity – in many schools of Chinese medicine, the mind is considered the root of *all* ill health. Practices such as meditation, mindfulness and Nei Gong have been developed within various cultures to help cultivate the mind and lead to good health. In Chinese medicine literacy, cultivation of the mind is sometimes referred to as She Shen (cultivation of mind), Yang Shen (conservation of mentality) or Tiao Shen (regulation of mind) and is thought to be a method of keeping healthy, both physically and mentally, by regulating the Shen (spirit) and therefore the Qi and the Jing (essence).

Many Chinese medicine classics write about regulating the mind as a way to preserve health and prevent disease. To regulate the mind is to quieten the mind. This refers to a state of mind that is relaxed yet engaged, free from excessive desires and emotionally stable. The regulation of one's consciousness and thoughts are imperative to the cultivation of mind and the ability to think clearly and reasonably. To help the mind to concentrate and focus, it is suggested that one must fix their attention to one thing at a time, which is not so easy within the engaging world that we live. Focusing on just one thing is thought to prevent the mind from being diverted and divided, which can lead to impairment and overstrain.

To further regulate the mind, it is important for the mind to relax as much as it works and vice versa – a healthy balance of Yin and Yang. Our Shen leads our Qi. When the mind is relaxed and clear, our Qi will accumulate and be focused. If the Shen is scattered, Qi will dissipate. Hobbies and activities are an excellent way to engage the mind and yet let it relax and forget about the stresses of everyday life. From the viewpoint of mind cultivation and health, a constant need for desires and material wealth can lead to illness by agitating the heart, which will also upset the mind. A pursuit of fame and recognition also leads to illness, as failure to meet unreachable goals may lead to sadness, grief and pensiveness.

> Temperance in the emotions can prolong life. (Gong Tingxian, Ming Dynasty, *Longevity and Life Preservation*)

Emotional stability is equally important to health preservation. Chapter 5 of the *Huang Di Nei Jing* (*Yellow Emperor's Inner Classic*) states: 'Overindulgence in the five emotions can create imbalance. Emotions can injure the Qi.' Emotions are a common, natural part of our daily lives, and to suppress them would be wrong. In order to keep our emotional states rational and in harmony, it is necessary to vent them properly, as the specific situation calls for. This is known as regulating the emotions. For instance, for the majority of the time, anger is a 'normal' feeling that can be perfectly harmless in small quantities. However, if one fails to recognise and sufficiently deal with the anger at the time, it can become excessive or suppressed. It will then become an endogenous pathogenic factor and lead to an upward rush of Qi. In Western medicine this may manifest as hypertension or even stroke in more severe cases. On the other hand, laughter and happiness have long been said to be beneficial to our health. This is also a view within Chinese medicine and health preservation. In recent times, Ding Fulu, an expert in Chinese health preservation, proposed that 'long life can be expected with a delightful mind… Laughter, which outweighs medicine, can supplement the brain, activate the Jing Luo, regulate Qi and Blood, and eliminate irritability' (cited in L. Zhanwen and M. Lieguang, *Health Preservation in Traditional Chinese Medicine*).

The concept of 'life is but an illusion' is, in my view, not simply to suggest that we are living in a made-up reality or that life is a dream – it could be interpreted that life is what we make of it. When we are feeling positive and happy, we notice and appreciate the good things around us. Our physical body relaxes, our breath becomes smoother and our Qi flows freely. In this state our minds are open. When we feel negative or in a bad mood, we focus only on the problems that we have and on the negative things surrounding us. Our body naturally tightens up and causes stagnation within both mind and body, we become close-minded and we see the worst in a given situation – I am sure that most of us have been in a bad mood, and it seems that one bad thing happens after another. Negative emotions can also have an effect on those around us; however, so can positive emotions. Positive outlooks on life can rub off on other people.

MASSAGE, ACUPUNCTURE AND MOXIBUSTION

The principles for health preservation are much the same as they would be for the treatment of disease. The difference however between promoting health and eliminating disease is that health preservation focuses on promoting the essential Qi, invigorating and regulating the Qi and Blood of the Zang Fu organs and building up the Wei (protective) and Ying (nutritive) Qi levels. Contrastingly, the treatment of disease focuses more on balancing the excess or deficiency of the Qi, Blood, Yin and Yang, and eliminating internal and external pathogens. Therefore, in practice, point selection and type of massage/needle manipulation in massage/acupuncture for health preservation will vary from those of a specific treatment. The number of points selected may be fewer, and the manipulations may be more moderate as to let the body subtly do its job.

The contraindications of massage or acupuncture for health preservation should be the same as those for the treatment of disease. Additionally, it may be unsuitable for those who are pregnant, or extremely weak, and any health issues should be dealt with through proper disease treatment before health maintenance is sought.

The following is a short list of meridian points that are commonly used in health promotion and preservation.

Zu San Li (St36) (足三里) (Figure 36.1) is one of the most important and widely used points and is a point preferred to promote health to the whole body. The great physicians of the past Sun Simiao and Hua Tuo recommended that this point be regularly stimulated (through pressure, needling or moxibustion) in order to maintain health and to prevent the body from becoming diseased and feeble. This is supported by its function to assist in the transformation and transportation functions of the Spleen (the sea of Blood and Qi), thus aiding the absorption of nutrients from the foods that we eat. This consequently has a positive effect on our immune system and benefits our Qi and strength. Furthermore, Zu San Li has a strong regulating function, enabling the body to tend towards the norm. For example, this point can be used clinically to treat both hypertension and hypotension by regulating Qi and Blood.

Note: Due to the ability of St36 to help raise Yang Qi, regular moxibustion on this point should be avoided in people under the age of 30, as this can cause insomnia, restlessness or headaches.

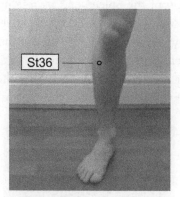

FIGURE 36.1: Zu San Li (St36)

He Gu (LI4) (合谷) (Figure 36.2) is an extremely popular point amongst acupuncturists, mainly for its function of alleviating pain. Due to the fact that the Yang Ming meridians are 'abundant in Qi and Blood', and this point is the Yuan source point of the Hand Yang Ming Channel, He Gu has the ability to move Qi and Blood strongly throughout the channels and encourage the movement of any stagnated Qi, particularly in the upper body. As stagnation is commonly seen as one of the main causes of disease within Chinese medicine, it would make sense that this point would be used in health preservation prescriptions in order to ensure the movement of Qi throughout the patient's body.

Note: This point is not to be used during pregnancy due to its strong action of moving Qi and Blood.

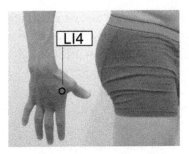

FIGURE 36.2: HE GU (LI4)

San Yin Jiao (Sp6) (三陰交) (Figure 36.3) is the crossing point of the three Yin meridians of the foot (K, Lv, Sp), and can therefore be used to treat all three organs. Its main function does indeed pertain to the harmonisation of the Spleen and its role in transportation and transformation; however, it is also very effective in promoting the free flow of Qi (by treating the Liver) and promoting longevity to the Kidneys by strengthening the Kidney Qi. Again, with the Spleen being the origin of the acquired Qi, fortifying the Spleen means the body's constitution will consequently be strengthened.

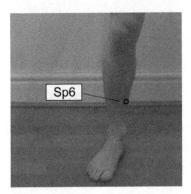

FIGURE 36.3: SAN YIN JIAO (SP6)

Yong Quan (K1) (涌泉) (Figure 36.4) is the lowest point of all meridians and is also the point that connects the body with the earth. Qi naturally rises, and as we become older the body's function in regulating the Qi and directing it downwards can become weaker. Clinically, this point is used to bring excessive Qi downwards, thus grounding the Qi and preventing disorders such as hypertension, dizziness and blurred vision. This point also has a strong effect on calming the mind and the emotions due to the close relationship of the Kidneys with the Heart. Needling this point can be quite sensitive – therefore it is recommended either to rub this point with enough force to create warmth, use moxibustion or visualise this point, and this should be done daily for health preservation.

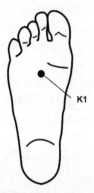

FIGURE 36.4: YONG QUAN (K1)

Guan Yuan (CV4) (關元) (Figure 36.5) tonifies the Kidney Qi, Yin and Yang and secures Jing. For this reason alone, this point is ideal for health promotion and preservation. Furthermore, it fortifies the Spleen and thus strengthens the overall constitution by invigorating the acquired Qi. Activating this area through visualisation can be powerful, and moxibustion is also a useful way to help activate it.

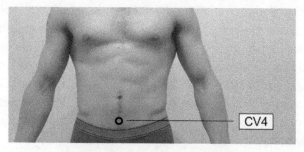

FIGURE 36.5: GUAN YUAN (CV4)

Qi Hai (CV6) (氣海) (Figure 36.6) primarily treats disorders of Qi and Kidney Yang. Sun Simiao once said that Qi Hai 'rules the Qi, enabling it to visit the five viscera'. As with Guan Yuan (CV4), this point tonifies the original Qi (pre-heaven Qi) and therefore connects with the five (or six) Zang organs and provides them with supplies of Qi. Consequently, stimulating this point can promote health to the overall Qi and thus the Zang organs.

Note: Indirect moxa can be applied to the lower Dan Tien area (CV4, CV5, CV6) for health preservation. A cone of loose moxa positioned on top of a slice of fresh ginger can be placed onto the lower Dan Tien regularly to promote health, invigorate Qi and Blood and promote digestion. This same method is also very effective on Zu San Li (St36) bilaterally. Moxibustion is said to have a significant function in regulating and strengthening the Spleen and Stomach (the origin of the acquired constitution and Qi).

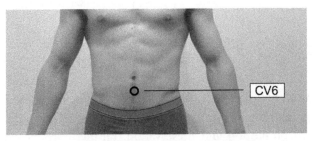

FIGURE 36.6: QI HAI (CV6)

Nei Guan (PC6) (內關) (Figure 36.7) is a very useful point for calming and harmonising the spirit. In clinical practice it is often used for any spirit disorders such as insomnia, poor memory and anxiety, due to its action of unbinding the chest and creating a smoother flow of Qi, and for this reason it is useful for maintaining a clear and calm mind. It also has a strong effect on harmonising the Stomach and Spleen due to its internal pathway descending through the three Jiaos, and it has a strong spiritual aspect of enabling the person to self-reflect. PC6 therefore is an excellent point for use in a health preservation prescription due to its effect on both mind cultivation and, indirectly, the body's acquired Qi.

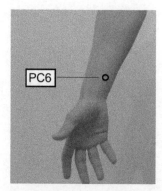

FIGURE 36.7: NEI GUAN (PC6)

Some classics also include Qu Chi (LI11) (曲池) in their lists of health preservation prescriptions due to the nature of the Yang Ming meridians being abundant in Qi and Blood. However, due to its strong function of clearing Heat and Fire within the body, this point can often be draining, and I do not believe it should be used on such a regular basis in case it causes deficiency. It is, however, a very effective point when used to reduce excess syndromes, such as in patients prone to hypertension. Shou San Li (LI10) (手三里) may be substituted instead for its energising effect on the upper limbs.

The choice of meridian points detailed above nicely reflects the other aspects of Yang Sheng in their functions: strengthen the acquired Qi (food therapy), calm the mind (cultivating the mind) and promote movement of Qi to prevent stagnation (Dao Yin exercises).

SUMMARY

The information in this and the previous chapter is only a very brief introduction to Chinese medicine and the Daoist concepts of Yang Sheng Fa, and has, I hope, generated interest for further reading on the subject. Although it seems almost impossible in this day and age to truly adhere to the ideals that the great physicians such as Sun Simiao wrote about, I strongly believe it is important for the practitioner to focus on their own health, as well as looking after their patients'. Yang Sheng Fa is a method to do this by incorporating many aspects of traditional and classical Chinese medicine. One's practice can inevitably benefit from the outcomes of self-cultivation.

37

ALCHEMY FOR MEN
Part 1
Tino Faithfull

Sit in the original emptiness to prevent desires from arising.
Ridding ourselves of desires helps us to bring about stillness.
Understanding this will enable all under Heaven to find peace.

Dao De Jing (Verse 37)

The set idea that women and men are supposed to train in the same way remains largely unquestioned in the world of the internal arts. Biological sex reflects distinct energetic properties, which should be taken into account in our training. The specificities of the female and male anatomies are particularly important in the context of alchemical training. Studying these specificities can help us understand the hurdles that practitioners of any gender will face throughout their training.[1]

This chapter looks at how men's energetic anatomy impacts their practice. Desires, especially those of a sexual nature, usually constitute the most significant obstacle for men. When desires take over, they disturb the essence (Jing). In order to lay strong foundations for internal alchemy, it is required that we go through a process of stilling the essence. This implies that we understand how essence moves inside

---

1   Please note that, throughout this chapter, the 'female' and 'male' categories are used as instances of two extremes that can be encountered on the gender compass (if there is such a thing!). I am aware that this approach simplifies the question of gender in ways that may be deemed problematic. However, such an oversimplification can help us understand the distinct energies of Yin and Yang and how they manifest inside the human body. Daoism would define gender as the balance of Yin and Yang in a person's nature. From this perspective, the study of gender involves the exploration of that balance and the acknowledgement of all the shades of grey that exist between these two poles.

the male body and how it reacts to external information. This is the study of Ming.

This chapter looks at the key differences between men and women and how these differences affect the movement of energy inside the human body. The next chapter focuses on the close relationship between essence and male desire.

NEI DAN GONG AND THE CONCEPT OF GENDER-SPECIFIC TRAINING

Nei Dan Gong, or internal alchemy, is traditionally considered the most advanced Daoist practice. There are many reasons for this. An obvious one – though easy to overlook – is that it takes a lot of body conditioning to be able to sit without any discomfort for long periods of time. In order to start working with the deeper aspects of our energy body (congenital meridians), the physical body must be open and free of any major blockages. We must also have started clearing and regulating the more superficial layers of our energy body (acquired meridians). The traditional approach would be to spend many years learning Qi Gong and Nei Gong. In doing so, we would build a strong foundation on both the physical and energetic planes. From there, the natural progression would be to start moving on to alchemy.

In the early stages of training in the Daoist arts, the practice is the same for both women and men. The first few years of training involve a lot of body conditioning – stretching and core work mainly. We also learn the various movements and sequences of the arts we have chosen to study. At this stage, the focus is very much on bringing ourselves to a state of balance. Our priority is to shed as many physical and emotional imbalances as possible. While it is possible to study Qi Gong and (to a certain extent) Nei Gong without looking too much into gender-specific training, this is definitely not the case for Nei Dan. The physiological differences that exist between women and men are the reflection of specific energetic blueprints. If we are to work with those blueprints, it is essential that we understand their nature. This must become part of our study.

NEI DAN GONG THEORY: THE CONCEPTS OF XING AND MING

When we start alchemy, there are two key concepts that need to be considered: Xing and Ming. Xing is generally translated as 'nature' and Ming as 'destiny'. Although not incorrect, these translations greatly reduce the meaning and scope of the two concepts, which are multi-layered; as such, they are probably better left untranslated. On a very superficial level, it could be said that Xing is mostly an expression of the mind while Ming relates primarily to the physical body. As shown in Figure 37.1, Xing is rooted in our Zhong Dan Tien (中丹田), or middle energy field, and Ming is rooted in our Xia Dan Tien (下丹田), or lower energy field.

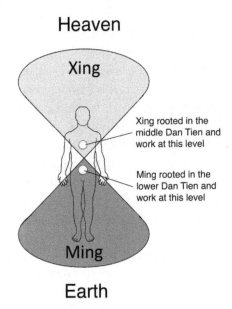

FIGURE 37.1: XING AND MING: THE TWO ASPECTS OF HUMAN EXISTENCE

Energetically, one of the key differences between women and men is how they relate to their lower and middle Dan Tien. Women are more connected to their middle Dan Tien, which means that they are naturally more in tune with the energy world. Men, on the other hand, tend to be more in line with their lower Dan Tien; as a result, they usually have a stronger connection to physicality.

Alchemy relies on a systematic process of transformation of various substances inside the human body. The three main substances that are involved in this process are Jing, Qi and Shen – or 'essence', 'energy' and 'spirit'. Daoism makes it clear that there is a natural progression that must be followed in order to achieve this process. Thus, we must first work on converting Jing to Qi. Only then can we start refining Qi to Shen and eventually Shen to Dao – so we can return to the 'unnamed' source. This process of conversion is shown in Figure 37.2.

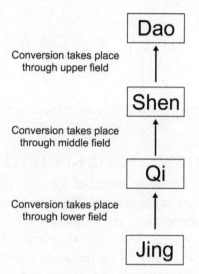

FIGURE 37.2: ALCHEMY: A PROCESS OF VIBRATIONAL TRANSFORMATION

Jing is anchored in the lower field and so belongs to the realm of Ming. Qi is anchored in the middle field and so belongs to the realm of Xing. Figure 37.3 provides a more visual description of these correlations.

As Figure 37.3 shows, the lower field ties us into physicality, while the middle field ties us into the energy realm, which is also the realm of emotions.

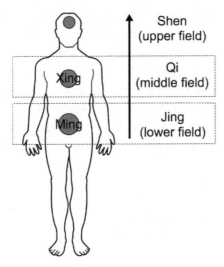

FIGURE 37.3: THE ENERGETIC MANIFESTATIONS OF XING AND MING

WOMEN AND MEN: SOME KEY DIFFERENCES

Daoism looks at the different realms of human experience – Jing, Qi and Shen – in terms of frequencies. The female energetic blueprint guarantees that women will be naturally more in tune with the frequency of their middle field (Qi). By contrast, the male energetic blueprint causes men to pick up the frequency of the lower field (Jing) much more easily. These specific predispositions give us a clue as to the main hurdles that practitioners of either gender will face in their training. In the context of alchemy, the main obstacle for women lies in the emotional realm. Women's privileged relation to the middle field makes them very attuned to their emotions. This also means that, at specific stages in their training, these emotions are likely to become disruptive and slow the progress of female practitioners. However, this hurdle only tends to become problematic at the stage of working with the middle field – which implies that a lot of work has already been done with the lower field.

Women have a tremendous advantage over men in that their affinity with the middle field causes them to be very receptive to the energy realm. For this reason, the early stage of converting Jing into Qi is usually fairly easy for them to achieve. This is not the case for men though. Their inherent energetic disposition can become an obstacle to their internal development, especially in the early days.

Being primarily rooted in physicality, they usually find it difficult to contact the energy realm. In other words, the key hurdle for men is the stage of converting Jing into Qi. This is partly because male Jing is programmed to stay in the region of the lower field. Female Jing, by contrast, is programmed to move up towards the chest. This energetic pattern is mirrored in the physiological signs that distinguish the female and male bodies.

It is usually accepted that, in both women and men, Jing is stored in the kidney area – which is true, but only partially so.[2] From there, Jing starts moving to another location in the body; and that location is different depending on biological determination. For women, Jing moves down the lower back and then up to the chest, following the lower section of the Xiao Zhou Tian, or small water wheel. Thus, female Jing is stored both around the kidneys and in the breasts. This explains why leakage of essence for women usually takes place around Shan Zhong (膻中), the heart centre.

From the kidney region, male essence follows the direction of the Du Mai, or governing meridian, which runs down the back. However, and unlike female essence, it does not want to go up again by following the Ren Mai, or conception meridian, which moves up the front of the body. Instead, male Jing is strongly attracted to Hui Yin, which corresponds to the centre of the perineum. From there, it moves to the testicles, where it is stored. Thus, male essence is stored around both the kidneys and the testicles. The perineum area is considered the main point of leakage for men's essence.

The natural movement of essence in the male body – and specifically its gathering in the lower abdomen – indicates that Ming is a key aspect for men to take into consideration in their training.

THE MULTIFACETED 'MING MATRIX'

In order to integrate Ming into our practice, we must first understand the meanings and implications of this term. Ming is a rather abstract,

---

2   There is often a tendency amongst scholars to capitalise the vital organs of the body, when approached from a Chinese medicine perspective. The only system I am familiar with is the traditional Daoist one – I have never studied modern medical systems. I only ever talk about the organs from a Daoist perspective. Therefore, I do not see a valid reason to capitalise the organs. This is a collection of essays on Daoism, after all, so there can be no confusion!

multi-layered concept that can only be grasped through theoretical study. The concept is further complicated by the fact that all its different meanings are somehow intertwined. Obviously, you can only look into each aspect of Ming separately before being able to comprehend the bigger picture. This pattern applies to many aspects of Daoism, as it normally takes a long time before you can grasp the 'basic' concepts in their entirety. You have to build your understanding as you go along, through a mix of research and first-hand practical experience.

One way of looking at Ming is that it describes your life path – your journey from birth to death (see Figure 37.4). This is where the notion of Ming as your individual 'fate' or 'destiny' originates from.

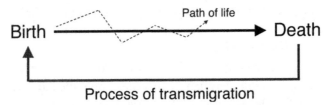

FIGURE 37.4: MING AS INDIVIDUAL LIFE PATH

To a great degree, your life path is an expression of the quality of the congenital essence that was given to you at birth. In other words, Ming is what determines how long your life is going to be. Here, we get a glimpse of the symbiotic relation between Ming and Jing. If we are not in line with our Ming, then our Jing will gradually become more and more depleted. Of course, the health of our Jing is also greatly dependent on external factors and personal life choices. This is where the study of Yang Sheng Fa – the art of nourishing our vitality – comes into play.

The character for Ming, shown in Figure 37.5, expresses several different ideas. The top part of the character is in the shape of a roof, which symbolises Heaven: this shows the close connection between Ming and Heaven. There are two more characters underneath: the one on the left shows a mouth speaking, and the one on the right evokes the notion of a contract.

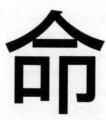

FIGURE 37.5: CHINESE CHARACTER FOR MING

Seen as a whole, the character for Ming expresses the idea of a contract or a mandate established between Heaven and each individual human being for the duration of their lifetime. The underlying idea is that the more we stick to this contract, the more pleasant the ride will be. If we can remain in line with our Ming, it is said that we will experience radiant health and longevity – providing we were not born with any major congenital weaknesses. However, the concept of Ming has more tangible ramifications within the human body. Ming is said to enter the body through a point called Ming Men, which is located between the two kidneys (see Figure 37.6). Ming Men can be translated as the 'gateway to Ming'. The passage of Ming through this point marks the transition from complete abstraction to something more tangible.

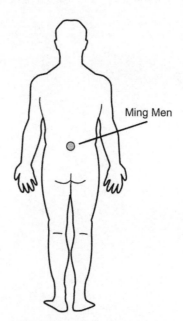

FIGURE 37.6: MING MEN LOCATION

From Ming Men, Ming descends towards Hui Yin and, as it moves towards physicality, it becomes our Jing. This is the process of materialisation of our essence. When it reaches Hui Yin, the Jing forms what is referred to as 'kidney water'. It is at this stage that our desires begin to form; these desires become the root of our key cravings. As it moves further down, Jing turns into bodily fluids. There is sometimes confusion as to the nature and function of Jing – especially with regard to the male body. In order to prepare ourselves for alchemy, it is essential that we understand how male Jing works. First, Jing is not semen, as is often believed. Jing is a vibration that manifests an energetic state that is very close to physicality; as such, it belongs to the realm of the 'almost tangible'. As explained above, the natural tendency of Jing is to move towards physicality. Once it manifests on the physical plane, it is not Jing any more. Instead, what we have is fluids. Some of the most relevant fluids with regard to alchemy training are semen (in the case of men) and menstrual blood (in the case of women). While those fluids are not Jing, their production – and subsequent waste – inevitably affects the energetic quality of our Jing.

The next chapter looks at the close relationship between Jing and male desire and explains why this relationship matters in the context of internal alchemy training.

38

ALCHEMY FOR MEN
Part 2
Tino Faithfull

In the previous chapter I explored the various meanings and implications of Ming in relation to alchemical training. In this chapter I look into the classical Daoist method for stilling the essence. This intensive practice requires that we spend a long period of time fully dedicated to Jing cultivation. In order to undertake this training, we need to adjust our lifestyle on many different levels. Throughout the chapter, I provide general advice as well as more specific guidelines on how to approach this traditional method.

JING AND MALE DESIRE

An overview of male Jing in relation to alchemy would not be complete without taking the sexual dimension into account. The relationship between Jing expense and sexual activity can be best understood by looking at what happens for men during orgasm. When women reach orgasm, they do not lose any bodily fluids. Every time men have an orgasm, their semen is wasted. Whether the semen is allowed out of the body or is retained inside at the point of ejaculation makes no difference whatsoever: it is lost all the same. In either case, the orgasm will have the same negative energetic imprint on the Jing. Women need not worry so much about regulating their sexual desires, which are not so detrimental to their practice and overall health. Men, on the other hand, must work on regulating their sexual desires, if they wish to lay appropriate foundations for Nei Dan Gong. Alchemical texts emphasise the need to 'still the Jing' prior to starting alchemy. In order to still the Jing, men must stop loss of fluids and quell their desires.

There is a direct connection between the pool of Jing in the perineum area (kidney water) and sexual desire. As men get sexually aroused, the Jing gathers around Hui Yin and starts moving into the length of the penis. The physical manifestation of this energetic movement is an erection. The surge of energy that takes place during an erection causes Hui Yin to move from the perineum area to the tip of the penis. Further stimulation will lead the Jing to move out of the penis, which manifests physically as an ejaculation of semen. The more regularly we ejaculate, the more our Jing will become accustomed to leaking out of the body. The natural movement of Jing from a congenital to an acquired state and its physical manifestation as bodily fluids is mapped out in Figure 38.1.

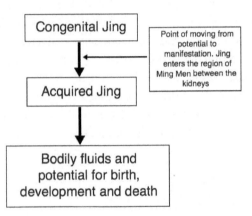

FIGURE 38.1: JING MOVEMENT FROM CONGENITAL TO ACQUIRED

As we expend our Jing, we move steadily towards decline. There is nothing abnormal about this. In fact, the most concise and, in my opinion, accurate definition of Jing would be 'what causes us to die' (slowly or not, depending on the circumstances). This natural bodily process is greatly accelerated by sexual activity though. According to classical Daoist teachings, the only way of curbing this great expense of essence is to go through a period of complete abstinence from sexual activity. This allows the acquired Jing to return to a state of stillness.

THE 'HUNDRED-DAY VIRGIN-BOY' TRAINING: LEARNING TO STILL THE JING

The classical technique for stilling the Jing is referred to as the 'hundred-day virgin-boy' training, which implies that we spend a hundred days without engaging in any sexual activity whatsoever. The idea underlying this practice is that it takes a hundred days for the acquired Jing to fully stabilise in the male body. Be aware that 'sexual activity' includes not only orgasm but also all kinds of sexual stimulation – which invariably cause the Jing to stir. For this reason, sexual imagery should be avoided too. The hundred-day training lays the foundation for the early stage of alchemy known as the 'firing process'. The firing process aims at 'reversing the course' by redirecting the movement of our Jing from the acquired realm back to the congenital realm. Instead of leaking out through Hui Yin, as it normally does, male Jing will now be recycled through the Xiao Zhou Tian (small water wheel) and the Chong Mai (central channel) (see Figure 38.2). While it's impossible to completely stop any leakage from taking place, the idea is to limit Jing depletion so it can be used for spiritual nourishment instead.

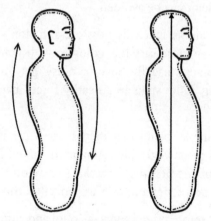

FIGURE 38.2: THE SMALL WATER WHEEL AND THE CHONG MAI

The firing process is initiated through a combination of controlled breathing and use of the muscles of the lower abdomen. However, this process can only be carried out successfully if we have managed to still our Jing and quieten our mind to a certain extent. Quelling desires – especially those of a sexual nature – is often a big challenge for men. To be honest, it is rather common for male practitioners to fail at this aspect of the training. If we cannot overcome our most deep-rooted desires, it is unlikely that we will manage to move past the very early stages of the alchemical process. Alchemy has the potential to transform our nature at a very deep level. Unfortunately, this formidable transformation cannot take place if the mind is constantly disturbed. A disturbed mind will automatically impact on the quality of our Jing. This is why we must also work on quieting the mind.

During the hundred-day training, it is also required that we adjust our lifestyle in order to encourage the stilling of the essence. Should you be interested in undertaking this training, here are a few simple guidelines to follow.

- Lead a quiet, simple life, away from the cacophony of the modern world.

- Stay away from large groups of people and trivial conversations.

- Avoid stress-inducing situations.

- Shun lurid, clamorous entertainment. Of course, it's fine to watch films; however, violence, action and pornography are obvious themes to be avoided.

- Stay at home as much as possible and don't go out unless it's absolutely necessary (i.e. going to work, buying groceries, etc.). If home is usually busy or noisy, get into the habit of taking long daily walks in a nearby forest, park or anywhere peaceful.

- Adopt a simple, bland diet that is based primarily on whole grains and green vegetables. Amaranth, millet, quinoa and rice are some of the best grain staples to rely on because of their balancing properties and calming effect on the mind.

- Cut out all meat, refined sugar, alcohol and coffee. Meat is here to be understood in its literal sense, namely as 'the flesh of an animal used for food'. Note: fish and shellfish are animals!

- Limit your dairy intake or, even better, cut it out completely.

- Avoid spices and strong flavours, as they stimulate the senses.

- In Ayurveda, allium plants are considered to fire up sexual desire – probably more than any other food. As such, it is probably best to stay away from them during your hundred-day training. Onions, garlic, leeks, shallots and chives are some of the most famous alliums.

In my experience, this diet is the most conducive to stilling the mind and building up the Jing for internal alchemy. For some people, these adjustments will feel like a drastic change; for others, they will be in the continuity of their lifestyle. Either way, you may encounter mental resistance, which, of course, should be treated as irrelevant. Soon enough, your mind will realise that all resistance is indeed futile!

RECONCILING TRAINING AND EVERYDAY COMMITMENTS

Now, there is the thorny question of who can realistically embark on such an intense and intensive training. Most people have a number of commitments they have to honour – work and family life being obvious instances. These commitments have to be taken into account, as there is a degree of personal responsibility involved. Be aware that the training does not get any less intense or less intensive after the hundred-day period of stilling the Jing. Going down the alchemical path – providing this is what you are interested in – is an all-consuming business. It is definitely not something you can do 'on the side', as you have to be ready to dedicate a lot of time to your training.

Should you start the hundred-day training if you don't have the time and space to commit to it fully? There is an argument for and there is an argument against – and I find them both to be valid for different reasons, so they are worth considering. As a teacher of the internal arts, I always try to be completely honest, as I feel there is a shocking lack of honesty in the modern world. People like to hear that anybody can achieve anything under any circumstances. That is simply not true. You cannot reach any significant stage of development in the internal arts without going through intensive periods of training. Yet, there are still people who think they can become proficient at those arts by merely attending a weekly class and not doing any personal training during the rest of the week.

In the current state of the world, values such as honesty and integrity are constantly trampled upon; they are not given the importance that they should have in everyday life. Everywhere corporations, banks and politicians thrive on the exploitation of poorer people. According to Daoism, the state of the macrocosm will always be reflected in the microcosm. No wonder, then, that so many people develop such a strong sense of entitlement. I have a problem with this culture of entitlement because it reveals a complete lack of integrity. This is why I choose to be as honest as I can.

I find 'no' to be a sensible answer to the aforementioned question. As far as alchemy is concerned, it is practically impossible to move beyond the very basic stages of internal development without dedicating several hours a day to your art. No less significant, how can the hundred-day training be realistically achieved without the time, space and focus that are required to still the essence and the mind? I am aware that this is probably not a very practitioner-friendly answer. The vast majority of practitioners (even the most dedicated ones) often do not have the required time and space to undertake a process as intensive as the hundred-day training. Usually, work is the main culprit. We have no other choice but to deal with the hurdles we encounter on the way. Thus, we must learn to reorganise what can be reorganised in our life, and what cannot be changed must be worked around.

There is another way of looking at the situation, which is perhaps more realistic and constructive for many people. It is technically possible to do the hundred-day training while still being actively involved in society. Obviously, the process will not yield the same results, but it can benefit other areas of your training – and this, in itself, should not be overlooked. Traditionally, Daoism did not advocate monastic life, away from society. This is why practitioners are actively encouraged to mingle and interact with non-practitioners. The argument is that there is no point cultivating your nature to a very high state if this state cannot be sustained in 'normal', everyday surroundings. Therefore, Daoism requires an alternation between sustained periods of retreat training and periods of immersion in society. Social immersion gives us an opportunity to use the surrounding chaos to consolidate our training and test our level of achievement. In the case of the hundred-day training, this is a real challenge, as this particular practice is clearly geared towards a retreat-type setting.

THE LIMITATIONS OF
NON-RECLUSIVE TRAINING

When doing the hundred-day training in a non-reclusive setting, most men will face the difficulty of keeping their sexual desires in check. Let's face it: we are constantly surrounded by stimuli of all sorts as soon as we step out the door. The glaring sexualisation of many areas of our lives is an added challenge. Besides, let us not underestimate the extent to which men are programmed to behave in certain ways. Biologically, the drive to reproduce is hardwired in our system – this is the congenital aspect of male programming. The acquired aspect of male programming is to do with social conditioning: from a very young age, men are encouraged to flirt constantly as a way of asserting their masculinity and their superiority over other men and women. One of the key functions of Daoist training is to help us identify this type of acquired programming and drop it. We must drop it because it is dumb.

Once you start the hundred-day training, you will no doubt marvel at your own conditioned behaviour. You may notice that you are constantly seeking to make eye contact with women and/or men around you. If you're sensitive enough, you may also feel the energetic effects of this ingrained habit on your state of mind. Once sexual energy starts stirring inside the body, the mind is disturbed and the Jing wants to move out of the body. This habit, which is very common in men, is particularly harmful, as it sets up a chain reaction, both physically and energetically. Once the mind is disturbed, it will not become quiet again until the accumulated acquired Jing has moved out of the body. In lay terms, your mind has now become used to the idea that there can be no peace until sexual release has taken place. This mental pattern is a clear sign that your willpower has become eroded.

THE FORCE OF HABITS

There is a direct relation between Ming and willpower. In Daoist thought, every vital organ has a spiritual blueprint that dictates various aspects of our nature and personality. Zhi is the spirit of the kidneys – as explained above, Ming relates to the kidneys. It is said that the quality of our Zhi controls our willpower. Thus, if our Zhi is weak, our willpower will be weak too. There are various factors – external and internal – that can cause our Zhi to fall out of balance. The most important factor to consider revolves around our deep-seated habits. Habits can refer to various types of attachments that manifest through repeated behaviours or mental processes.

The integration into your psyche of a pattern that has been presented to you as normal over a long period of time can turn into a deep-seated habit – flirting being a really good example. The mechanism that underlies such habits is usually unconscious. Social, political and educational types of conditioning inculcate automatic thought processes in individuals. Blaming 'the immigrants', 'the refugees' or poorer people for everything that is wrong in your country is a powerful, if topical, example of this type of conditioning. Do you find yourself constantly blaming immigrants for stealing jobs? Stop it. It's bad for your willpower!

On the most extreme end of the 'habit spectrum' are addictions. Addiction-type habits are particularly harmful as they drain our Jing very quickly. Common addictions include drugs, alcohol, food and – the most relevant one for most men – sex. Porn addiction, as common as it is, is a real issue, as it completely dissolves your willpower. There is a crucial misunderstanding around willpower and how it works. Willpower is usually considered to be a form of control deliberately exerted with the mind in order to restrain one's impulses. This is not the Daoist way, though.

HOW TO DEVELOP WILLPOWER

It is virtually impossible to get away from the wealth of stimuli that pervades society; that is the nature of everyday life. If we decide to undertake the hundred-day training while remaining socially active, we will be under constant pressure from the desires of the acquired mind. When those desires become too overwhelming, as they will, there are two choices: we can either give in or resist. If we give in to our desires, the training is over. If we choose to resist them over an extended period of time, we will end up burning up our Jing instead of stilling it. The resistance that arises when our desires start stirring up also hinders the development of our willpower. Too much resistance to our desires can manifest as nocturnal emissions, but not always. This is nothing to worry about though, especially if you're doing the non-reclusive version of the training. If nocturnal emissions occur, it is not required to start the training all over again. Leaking semen is definitely not a sign of failure and it is still worth carrying on with the process.

In everyday society, it is usually accepted that real willpower can only be achieved through ongoing mental struggle and resistance. Nothing could be further from the truth. From a Daoist perspective, willpower can only be cultivated by getting rid of the things that are directly weakening it; thus, it cannot be tackled in an upfront manner. Once the mental patterns impeding it are shed, willpower will arise on its own. As explained above, our willpower is weakened by deep-seated habitual patterns. The more we can shed those habits, the stronger our willpower will become. Shedding our habitual patterns can be done through a combination of external and internal methods. The sitting constitutes the internal method: by doing nothing, we allow the mind to reach stillness. This stage of alchemical training is called Zuo Wang – 'sitting and forgetting'. However, the internal method is often not enough on its own, especially in the early stages of alchemical training.

The external method involves a thorough work of introspection and self-analysis. This means that we have to be as honest with ourselves as we can as far as our desires and obsessive mental patterns are concerned. We must first identify our own individual pattern of habitual conditioning so we can let go of the acquired mind. Very often, placing your awareness on a negative process (whether it is physical or mental) is enough for it to start dissolving (the process, not the awareness – although dissolving the awareness sounds good too!). Awareness is the key word when it comes to shedding the acquired mind: every time we bring an unconscious pattern into our field of awareness, we move closer to our true nature. When we manage to sit in relative (or, even better, complete) stillness, the same work of dissolving our acquired nature takes place. Once we have laid the foundation, the most efficient way of quelling our desires is the sitting itself. As implied in the *Dao De Jing*, we 'sit in the original emptiness to prevent desires from arising'.[1]

To conclude this extensive reflection on alchemy for men, I would like to re-emphasise the fact that it is possible to do the hundred-day alchemical training while being socially active. People have done it

---

1   See the full quote at the beginning of the previous chapter.

before and found it beneficial to their practice in lots of ways. However, shorter periods of intensive Jing cultivation seem to give much better results – especially in the early stages of training. In my opinion, four weeks is an ideal length of time, as it is long enough to start the process of quelling desires while not being long enough to burn up significant amounts of Jing as a result of mental resistance. This four-week process will be especially beneficial if repeated several times in the first few years of training. I would recommend doing it once a year until you can find the right time and space to undertake the hundred-day training in more appropriate conditions.

My first periods of intensive Jing work were done in situations where I was socially involved, because I had no other choice at the time. I found that those periods brought me a lot of mental focus and increased my vitality significantly; these are important signs of progress for alchemical training. This is all part of building a strong foundation for our practice. Only later did I find myself in the right position to undertake the full version of the hundred-day training in ideal conditions. The good news is that it did not feel like starting the process all over; it felt more like building on previous attempts at stilling the Jing. Consolidating and stilling the essence is a gradual process that can only be achieved over a long period of time – as such, it is a genuine form of Gong Fu.

The truth is that there is no fast track to internal development.

The ultimate function of Jing cultivation is not to stop all leakage of essence. Rather, the aim is to develop as much awareness as possible. The simple fact of maintaining a very high degree of awareness for a full hundred days is a large step in the right direction. Valuable benefits can be gained from the training if we can stay very aware for long periods of time (as opposed to, say, obsessively focusing on preventing nocturnal emissions). Awareness is the exact opposite of mental struggle; it is the key for developing willpower and everything else in life. If we can sustain awareness for long enough, all resistance and weakness will eventually dissolve. The acquired layers of our mind will fade and our true congenital nature will begin to shine through.

GLOSSARY OF PINYIN TERMS

This is a glossary of Pinyin Chinese terms used within this book as well as within previous titles written by the author Damo Mitchell. It can be confusing coming into the Daoist arts and encountering so many Chinese names and words. The fact is that direct translation into English can be difficult with many of these terms, but we have attempted to make them as clear and concise as possible.

Ba Gua 八卦: The Daoist theory of the eight key energies of the universe. This is the basic tenet of the *Yi Jing* as well as countless other aspects of the tradition.

Bai Hui 百會 (DU20): An acupuncture point situated on top of the head. Translated as meaning 'hundred meetings'. In esoteric Daoism it is also the point where numerous spirits converge and the point where the Chong Mai extends upwards out of the body.

Bi Yan Hu 碧眼胡: The 'blue-eyed foreigner'; a name for Bodhidharma, the patriarch of Chan Buddhism within China.

Chan 禪: The form of Buddhism commonly taught within China. A combination of Buddhist and Daoist theory.

Da Zhou Tian 大周天: 'Large heavenly cycle'; also known as the 'large water wheel of Qi'. This is the primary circulation of energy out of the body, which can be achieved through consistent Nei Gong or Nei Dan training.

Dan 丹: The Dan is the 'elixir' that is sought out through alchemical training within the Daoist tradition. It is often depicted as red and likened to the ore of cinnabar.

Dan Tien 丹田: Usually refers to the lowest of the three main 'elixir fields', though there are three main Dan Tien within the body. The primary function of the lower Dan Tien is the conversion of Jing to Qi as well as the moving of Qi throughout the meridian system.

Dao 道: The nameless and formless origin of the universe. Daoism is the study of this obscure concept, and all internal arts are a way of experientially understanding the nature of Dao.

Dao De Jing 德道经: The 'virtue of following the way'. The classical text of Daoism written by the great sage Laozi. Also written as *Tao Te Ching*.

Dao Yin 導引: 'Guiding and pulling' exercises; these are the ancient exercises developed by the shamanic Wu people to purge the energy body of pathogenic energies.

Dao Zang 道藏: The Daoist canon of classical writings, which includes over 1400 pieces of scripture.

De 德: The congenital manifestation of the transient emotions. De is born from deep within the true human consciousness, which is usually buried beneath the various layers of the acquired mind.

Ding 鼎: The 'cauldron' of Daoist Nei Dan. This is a location within the energy body where two energetic substances are being combined. Named after the Ding that sits within most Daoist temples.

Dui 兑: One of the eight trigrams of Daoist Ba Gua theory. Its energetic manifestation is metaphorically likened to a lake, although Dui does not directly mean lake.

Feng Shui 风水: 'Wind and water'; this is the Daoist study of environmental energies and the influence of the macrocosm upon the human energy system and consciousness.

Fu 符: The magical talismanic drawings of the ancient Daoists. The skilled practitioner of magical Daoism could draw Fu to heal sickness, curse people or perform countless other functions. An almost extinct art in modern times.

Gen 艮: One of the eight trigrams of Daoist Ba Gua theory. Its energetic manifestation is likened to that of a mountain.

Gong 功: The attainment of a high-level skill within any art. To truly attain Gong took a lifetime of dedicated study, especially within the internal arts.

Gua 卦: 'Trigram'; these are the eight sacred symbols that make up Daoist Ba Gua theory. They are a way to conceptualise the various vibrational frequencies of the energetic realm and how they interact.

Hou Tian 後天: The 'post Heaven' state that we exist within according to Daoist thought.

Hui Yin 會陰 (CV1): 'Meeting of Yin' is an acupuncture point located at the perineum. It is named after the fact that it is situated within the most Yin area of the human body.

Hun 魂: 'Yang soul'; the ethereal soul that continues to exist after our death. It is usually housed within the Liver.

Hundun 混沌: A term generally translated as referring to 'original chaos'. Within Daoist philosophy it refers to a state that lay dormant within the centre of human consciousness as well as an aspect of the process of creation. It is also the name of a stance used within female-specific Nei Gong training.

Ji Ben Qi Gong 基本气功: 'Fundamental energy exercises'; the primary exercises taught within the Lotus Nei Gong School of Daoist Arts.

Jing 精: The lowest vibrational frequency of the three main energetic substances of man. Usually translated as meaning 'essence' and often misunderstood as being human sexual fluids.

Jing Gong 精功: 'Essence exercises'; the technique of building up and refining our Jing.

Jing Jin 經筋: Lines of connective tissue that run throughout the body. These lines serve as 'riverbeds' for the flow of Qi that runs through the meridian system. The term is generally translated as meaning 'tendon collaterals', but it is the author's opinion that in many respects this term is actually referring to lines of fascia.

Jing Luo 经络: The human meridian system that is made up of numerous energetic pathways that regulate the body and transport Qi to and from our organs and tissues.

Kan 坎: One of the eight trigrams of Daoist Ba Gua theory, which is usually likened to the energetic manifestation of water. It is especially important within the practice of Nei Dan.

Kun 坤: One of the eight trigrams of Daoist Ba Gua theory. Its energetic manifestation is usually likened to that of the planet.

Kun Lun Shan 崑崙山: A mythical mountain within Daoist legend, which was said to reach up into the Heavens.

Lao Gong 勞宮 (PC8): An acupuncture point situated in the centre of the palm. Its name means 'palace of toil' due to it being on the human hand, which carries out a lot of physical work. Within Daoism they also know this point to be very important in venting heat from the heart and so it is rarely at rest. It is a very important point in Qi Gong practice, as it regulates the internal temperature and also allows us to emit Qi in practices such as external Qi therapy.

Laozi 老子: The great sage. The 'original Daoist' who wrote the *Dao De Jing*. Supposedly, he left this text with a border watchman when he retreated into hermitage in the western mountains of China.

Li 離: One of the eight trigrams of Daoist Ba Gua theory. Its energetic manifestation is usually likened to fire. It is especially important to understand within the context of Nei Dan training.

Liang Yi 兩儀: The collective name for Yin and Yang. It is literally translated as meaning the 'two poles'.

Long Dao Yin 龍導引: 'Dragon Dao Yin'; a set of four sequences based upon the preliminary training methods from the martial style of Baguazhang. They twist the spine and open the joints to assist with the energetic purging process.

Lu 爐: The 'furnace' of Daoist Nei Dan. This is the place within the body where expansion is created, which generates heat. This heat is then usually added to the Ding in order to create alchemical change.

Ming 命: Your predestined journey from life to death. It is usually translated as meaning 'fate', but this really does not explain the true meaning of the term.

Ming Men 命门 (GV4): An acupuncture point in the lower back that is very important in Nei Gong practice. This point is referred to several times in this book, and serious internal arts practitioners should work very hard to awaken the energy in this area of their meridian system.

Nei Dan 内丹: The Daoist form of alchemical meditation usually associated with the northern sects of Daoism. Through working with various energetic and spiritual substances within the body, the practitioner seeks states of transcendence and, ultimately, immortality.

Nei Gong 内功: The process of internal change and development that a person may go through if they practise the internal arts to a high level.

Nei Jing Tu 内经图: The 'chart of the inner landscape'; one of two important alchemical charts carved into a courtyard wall of the 'white cloud monastery' in Beijing.

Nu Dan 女丹: The practice of 'women's alchemy'. A slightly different process exists for women due to the nature of their energetic systems.

Po 魄: The 'Yin soul' that dies with the human body. Largely connected to our physical senses, the Po resides in the lungs.

Pu 樸: 'Simplicity'; often likened to being like an 'uncarved block'. The ideal state of mind according to the Daoist tradition. This has much to do with shedding the layers of the acquired mind, which pull you away from existing in a simple state.

Qi 氣: 'Energy'; a term that is often difficult to translate into English. In Nei Gong theory it is an energetic vibration that transports information through the energy system.

Qi Gong 氣功: Usually gentle exercises that combine rhythmic movements with breathing exercises to shift Qi through the body. The term means 'energy exercises', although it is sometimes translated as meaning 'breathing exercises'.

Qi Hai 氣海 (CV6): An acupuncture point that sits in front of the lower Dan Tien. Its name in English means 'sea of Qi', as it is the point from where Qi is generated and where it flows from. Like water returning to the sea in rivers and streams, Qi returns to the lower Dan Tien when it circulates in the 'small water wheel of Qi'.

Qian 乾: One of the eight trigrams of Daoist Ba Gua theory. Its energetic manifestation is usually likened to the movements of Heaven.

Ren 人: Within Daoism, Ren is 'humanity'. Humanity sits between Heaven and Earth and is a reflection of their fluctuations and movements. Ren is nourished by Earth and stimulated to development through the actions of Heaven.

San Bao 三寶: The 'three treasures' of man, which are Jing, Qi and Shen.

Shen 神: The energy of consciousness. It vibrates at a frequency close to that of Heaven. It is manifested within the body as a bright, white light.

Shen Gong 神功: This is the arcane skill of working with the substance of consciousness. Within Daoism it is said that a skilled Shen Gong practitioner can manipulate the very energy of the environment.

Shen Xian 神仙: The 'Heavenly immortal' is essentially full realisation of the possibility of spiritual immortality, which is the final goal of Daoist Nei Dan.

Sun 巽: One of the eight trigrams of Daoist Ba Gua theory. Its energetic manifestation is usually likened to that of the wind.

Taiji 太极: A Daoist concept of creation that can be translated as meaning the 'motive force of creation'.

Taiyi 太一: The 'great pole' of Daoist philosophy is the single point of union that moves out of stillness. It is also the name of a standing posture utilised in advanced female-specific Nei Gong training.

Tian 天: 'Heaven'; not to be mistaken for the Christian concept of Heaven, this refers to the vibrational frequency of the macrocosm. Within the microcosm of the body Heaven is used to refer to human consciousness metaphorically.

Tian Gan 天干: The 'Heavenly stems' is a model of the Yin and Yang divisions that take place within the Wu Xing within the Heavenly realm.

Tian Gui 天癸: An energetic component involved in the formation of menstrual blood for women. The term is often translated as meaning 'Heavenly Water'.

Tui Na 推拿: A form of Chinese medical massage that means 'push and grasp'.

Wu 巫: The shamanic Wu were the historical ancestors of the Daoists. They served as medicine men, bringers of rain and general mystics to the ancient tribes of China.

Wu Shen 五神: The 'five spirits'; the collective name for the Shen, Hun, Yi, Zhi and Po.

Wu Wei 無為: The act of 'non-governing'. An important philosophical concept within the Daoist tradition. This term is often misunderstood to mean that Daoists should 'do' nothing and thus are essentially lazy.

Wu Xing 五行: The five elemental energies that are an important part of Daoist creation theory, psychology and medicine.

Wu Xing Qi Gong 五行气功: 'Five Element energy exercises'; they are an important part of the Lotus Nei Gong School of Daoist Arts syllabus.

Wuji 无极: The Daoist concept of non-existence. The blank canvas upon which reality is projected and an important part of Daoist creation philosophy.

Xian Tian 先天: The 'before Heaven' congenital state that is all important within Nei Dan training.

Xin-Yi 心意: 'Heart-Mind'; this is the framework with which we attempt to understand the various aspects of human consciousness. Originally a Buddhist concept, it was absorbed into Daoist teachings.

Xing 性: Your 'nature'; this is the expression of the various energetic and spiritual components of consciousness.

Xiu Zhen Tu 修真图: The 'chart of cultivating perfection'; a highly influential chart within the Daoist alchemical tradition.

Xiwangmu 西王母: The 'holy mother of the west' is a Daoist immortal and deity associated with the power of the western Heavens, prosperity and immortality. She is often the patron deity of many female Daoist practitioners. She is often associated with the seven star constellation.

Yang 陽: The Daoist philosophical extreme of movement, masculinity and action. One of the two great points that is required to manifest existence.

Yang Qi 阳氣: Within Chinese medicine this refers to our internal Qi, which moves out towards the surface of the body and the congenital meridians. Within Nei Dan theory it can also refer to the state of energy prior to its movement into the realm of existence.

Yang Sheng Fa 养身法: Literally 'life nourishing principles', this is the Daoist practice of living healthily, which should be studied alongside all internal arts.

Yi 意: 'Intention' or 'awareness'; an important element of human consciousness to cultivate in Nei Dan training.

Yi Jing 易经: The 'classic of change'; an ancient Daoist text that is based upon Ba Gua theory. It is commonly written as *I Ching*.

Yin 陰: The Daoist philosophical pole of stillness, femininity and quietude. One of the two poles required in order for existence to come into being.

Yin Qi 阴氣: Our internal Qi, which moves inwards to nourish the organs of the body. It can also be used within alchemical theory to describe the movement of Wuji as it coalesces around the condensed energy of Yang Qi.

Yin Tang 印堂: A meridian point situated between the eyebrows. Translated as the 'hall of impression', it is often equated with the spiritual third eye of the Eastern arts.

Yong Quan 涌泉 (K1): An acupuncture point on the base of the foot that means 'bubbling spring'. This is the main point through which earth energy is drawn into the body.

Yuan Jing 元精: The original essence that exists prior to the beginning of the movement of the acquired essence. It is said to reside in the space between the Kidneys.

Yuan Qi 元氣: The original state of Qi prior to its movement into the acquired realm.

Yuan Shen 元神: The original state of human psyche prior to the movement from the congenital to the acquired. It exists as a brilliant white light within the space of the human Heart-Mind.

Yuan Xi 元息: 'Original breath'; the breath of life that is passed down into existence from Dao. Yuan Xi is an expression of the movement of Yuan Qi.

Zang Fu 脏腑: The collective name for the Yin and Yang organs of the body.

Zhen 震: One of the eight trigrams of Daoist Ba Gua theory. Its energetic manifestation is often likened to thunder.

Zhen Ren 真人: The 'true person' of Daoism is a high-level state of attainment possible through alchemical cultivation of the inner state.

Zhi 志: An element of human consciousness that is directly linked to the state of our Kidneys. The nearest translation in English is 'willpower'.

Zhuangzi 莊子: An important sage within the Daoist tradition. Zhuangzi was known for his humour and the fact that he poked fun at almost every aspect of life.

Zi Bao 子胞: The 'child container' is the Uterus as well as the energetic matrix associated with this physical organ within the female body.

Zi Fa Gong 自發功: The process of releasing spontaneous energetic movements through the body. This happens as stagnant energetic pathogens are released and the body begins to return to some kind of order.

Ziran 自然: The Daoist philosophical concept of acting in harmony with nature and returning to an original state.

Zuo Wang 坐忘: This can be translated as meaning 'sitting and forgetting'. This is the entering of the silent state during Daoist meditation.

ABOUT THE CONTRIBUTORS

Damo Mitchell began his studies of the Eastern arts at the age of four, and these practices have continued throughout his life. He is the technical director of the Lotus Nei Gong School of Daoist Arts and the author of several books published by Singing Dragon. He currently lives in Portugal but maintains schools in the UK, Sweden, America and Canada.

Donna Pinker studied Chen and Yang-style Taijiquan for many years before joining the Lotus Nei Gong School in 2008. Since this time she has studied the internal arts with Damo Mitchell and other senior teachers in the school. She now runs her own classes in Bristol, UK, as well as being a qualified Shiatsu practitioner.

Ellie Talbot is a long-time student of Taijiquan and Qi Gong under various teachers including Damo Mitchell and Steve Galloway. She continues her studies in courses across Europe as well as assisting with teaching classes in Lotus Nei Gong's North Wales classes.

Kulsoom Shah trains in the American branch of Lotus Nei Gong with Damo Mitchell. She is a student of Nei Gong with a background in Chen-style Taijiquan. Alongside this she studies Chinese medicine at university level in America.

Lauren Faithfull has been studying Nei Gong and the internal martial arts with the Lotus Nei Gong School for many years. She also teaches her own classes and courses alongside her partner Tino Faithfull in various places, including France, the UK, Portugal and America.

Linda Hallett is a Qi Gong teacher within the Lotus Nei Gong School as well as an acupuncturist. She runs a clinic in Shropshire (UK) and continues her studies in Taijiquan and the internal arts with Damo Mitchell, Steve Galloway and Paul Mitchell in various locations around Europe.

Paul Mitchell is Damo Mitchell's father and his first teacher of the martial arts. Paul has studied Yang Taijiquan (including variations on the style) for many years as well as Nei Gong and Shotokan Karate-Do. He teaches classes in Somerset, UK, as well as running courses for Lotus Nei Gong in various parts of Europe.

Richard Agnew started his martial arts studies at a young age. In 2005 he met Grandmaster Wong Kiew Kit and this led him deeper into Qi Gong and then acupuncture, which he studied at the College of Integrated Chinese Medicine in Reading, UK. In 2013 he became a student of Damo Mitchell and now continues his studies within the school. He runs his acupuncture clinic in Surrey, UK.

Rob Aspell came from a background of Wing Chun and then moved into Chinese medicine, including herbs, acupuncture and Tui Na massage. He now runs a busy clinic in North Wales as well as teaching alongside Damo Mitchell at the Xian Tian College of Daoist Medicine in the South of the UK.

Roni Edlund is Damo's partner and has been studying the Daoist arts full time for many years. She teaches Taijiquan, Baguazhang and Nei Gong within Lotus Nei Gong as well as within her own school, the Lotus Moon School of Spiritual Arts, which is specifically for women. She is also the author of the book *Daoist Nei Gong for Women*, which is published by Singing Dragon.

Seb Smith is one of the longest-standing members of the Lotus Nei Gong School. He has studied Yang Taijiquan and Nei Gong with Neil Lodge of the Cardiff branch as well as spending extended periods of time in retreat with Damo Mitchell in Europe and Asia. He is also a qualified medical doctor, which helps to inform the medical sides of his Daoist study.

Tino Faithfull is one of the senior teachers of the Lotus Nei Gong School of Daoist Arts. He studies Taijiquan, Nei Gong, Baguazhang and alchemy with Damo Mitchell and has spent extended periods in retreat with him. He runs his own school of Daoism as well as teaching with Damo. He is currently focusing on teaching Nei Gong methods internationally.

INDEX

acquired
  aspect of male
    programming 291
  connection to Ming 123
  Jing 67, 112, 286–7, 291
  meridians 113, 277
  mind 22, 25, 27, 47–50,
    52–3, 110, 112–13,
    125–6, 130, 136, 187,
    189–90, 239–40, 292–4
  nature 25, 112, 123,
    125–8, 131, 134,
    136–7, 211, 233, 293
  Qi 60, 113, 264, 272–5
  self 144, 235
  Shen 113
  spirit 115
  see also Hou Tian
acupuncture
  affecting emotional state 50
  Bai Hui point 238
  concentration and focus
    as key to 264
  for health preservation 270–5
  Ming Men point 69
  treating worms 30–4
addictions
  feeding worm 34
  as habits 30, 292
  rectifying 240–3
Air 88
alchemy
  about creating movement
    within channels 114–15
  aim of 222
  alchemical circulation 21
  alchemical conversion
    58, 64, 115, 117
  alchemical Daoism
    energy of emotions 45
    focus on body 186
    Fu 38
    and mindfulness 29
    schools 211
    Shen 44, 152–3
    spirits to regulate 218
    theory 118
  alchemical elixir 18, 27,
    55–6, 59, 109–10

alchemical interaction of
  Fire and Water 25
alchemical language
  of channels 113
  Heart and Kidneys in 24
  as occasionally
    confusing 25
  pineal gland in 151
alchemical meditation
  Ding and Lu in 11
  effective sitting
    practice 41–4
  as form of meditation 111
  Li and Kan in 26–7
  meaning given to Qi 42
  Yin and Yang in 26–7
alchemical model 17–19, 21
alchemical process
  'cooking' substances 61–2
  within Ding 13–14
  moving past early
    stages of 288
  powers brought together
    for completion of 13
  'receiving three strikes
    of thunder' 128
  Yin and Yang in 13
alchemical production of
  Heaven and Earth 27
alchemical reaction
  Heart and Kidneys 24
  within lower abdominal
    region 14
alchemical texts 57–8, 128,
  140–1, 174, 195, 285
  Daoist internal 111, 115
  division into two schools
    of thought 89
  'firing process' 287
  as form of esoteric
    Daoism 118
  hundred-day training
    287–92, 294
  and immortality 117,
    143, 221
  importance of respiration 56
  important fires within
    body for 171
  and Jing 284–5, 289
  main obstacle for women 280

meaning of 45–6
for men 276–94
patience and perseverance
  for 65
potential to transform human
  nature at deep level 288
as process of vibrational
  transformation 279
Qi within 60
stages before entering
  emptiness 111
symbolic representation 195–6
Xing and Ming, when
  starting 278
Zuo Wang stage 293
see also internal alchemy
alignment
  common mistakes 255
  correct 254–5
  knee pain 254, 259–60
  other structural issues
    'dropped' arches 258–9
    tight iliotibial band/
      tensor fasciae latae 257
    vastus medialis
      weakness 254
    weak gluteal muscles 255
  resolving mistakes 256–7
'all-seeing eye' 152–4
An Mo see Tui Na
apathy 103, 105, 218
argument phase of sitting
  practice 49–50
attachments 25, 28–9, 31–2,
  208, 219, 240–3

Bai Gui 216
Bai Hui 238
Bai Hui fire 135
Bi Gu 35–6
bitter foods 177–8, 182
Blake, W. 195
Blood 178, 213, 264, 267,
  269–71, 274–5
boredom, during sitting
  practice 51–3
breath
  absorbing environmental
    energy through 213
  controlled use of 12